Educatio
Southend
Westcliff-
Tel: Tel

Staff Nurse Survival Guide

Staff Nurse Survival Guide
Essential questions and answers
for the practising staff nurse

Edited by John Fowler

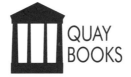

Quay Books Division, MA Healthcare Ltd, St Jude's Church, Dulwich Road,
London SE24 0PB

British Library Cataloguing-in-Publication Data
A catalogue record is available for this book

© MA Healthcare Ltd 2005
ISBN 1 85642 233 X

All rights reserved. No part of this publication may be reproduced, stored in a retrieval system
or transmitted in any form or by any means, electronic, mechanical, photocopying, recording
or otherwise, without prior permission from the publishers

Printed by Cromwell Press, Trowbridge, Wiltshire

Contents

Contributors	ix
Introduction	xiii

Chapter 1: How do I deal with emergencies?   1

❖ What do I need to know about cardiorespiratory arrest?	1
❖ How do I carry out basic life support?	4
❖ What do I need to know about haemorrhage?	10
❖ How do I recognise and assess significant haemorrhage?	12

Chapter 2: How do I deal with the unexpected?   21

❖ How do I deal with difficult questions?	21
❖ How do I deal with complaints?	23
❖ How do I deal with aggressive patients or relatives?	25
❖ What is involved in incident reporting?	27
❖ What are my responsibilities in reporting malpractice	29
❖ What can I do about bullying within the organisation?	31
❖ What do I do if a patient wants to self-discharge?	33
❖ How do I deal with MRSA?	34

Chapter 3: What principles do practical nursing skills involve?   39

❖ What is the essential role of the nurse?	39
❖ What are the principles of caring for patients with wound drains?	40
❖ How do I look after a nasogastric or gastric tube?	42
❖ What is the nursing management of intravenous therapy?	45
❖ What is involved in catheterisation and catheter care?	47
❖ What is a syringe driver?	52
❖ How do I monitor central venous pressure?	53
❖ What do I need to know about different wound dressings?	54
❖ What does an aseptic technique involve?	57
❖ What are the principles of preparing patients for tests and investigations?	58
❖ How can I promote continence?	64
❖ What are the common signs and symptoms of a urinary tract infection?	65
❖ What do I need to know about pressure ulcers?	66
❖ How do I help my patients meet their nutritional needs?	69

v

Chapter 4: How do I discharge patients or refer them to other services?   73

- How do I refer patients to the community services?   73
- How do I refer patients to the multidisciplinary team?   75
- How do I refer patients to specialist nurses?   76

Chapter 5: What are the principles of patient medication?   79

- What is the nurse's role in drug administration?   79
- What legislation governs medications and are there other national documents that guide us in this practice?   80
- How do drugs work?   82
- What are the principles of safe practice for giving medication?   90
- What do I need to know about drug calculations?   94
- What are the routes of drug administration?   100
- What are the ethical issues in drug administration?   106
- How can I avoid drug errors?   107
- What are the alternative and new initiatives in drug administration?   109

Chapter 6: How do I look after a student?   115

- What is the role of the mentor?   115
- What is involved in teaching a student?   121
- What is involved in assessing a student?   126

Chapter 7: How do I work with others?   131

- How do I work with others and become part of the team?   131
- How do I deal with experienced healthcare assistants?   134
- What am I meant to do on a ward round?   134

Chapter 8: How do I look after myself?   137

- How do I manage my time?   137
- How do I get to grips with working unsocial hours?   139
- What should I expect from clinical supervision?   140
- What do I need to know about the research process?   140
- What is involved in professional development?   142
- How can I develop my professional practice?   145
- What sort of post-registration course should I do?   147
- What are CAT points and APAs?   148
- What is involved in reflective practice?   151
- How do I prepare for an interview?   153

Chapter 9: What is my role in dealing with grief, bereavement and palliative care?   157

- How do I talk with patients, relatives and carers?   157
- How do I contact relatives/carers following a death?   158
- What if I'm involved in caring for a terminally ill child?   161
- How do I care for the patient's body after death?   163
- How do I manage pain in palliative care?   164
- What are the causes of pain in advanced cancer?   166
- What is the analgesic three-step ladder?   167
- What other ways are there of managing pain in palliative care?   168
- How do I manage nausea and vomiting in palliative care?   169
- How do I manage intestinal obstruction in palliative care?   172
- How do I manage constipation in palliative care?   173
- How do I manage dyspnoea in palliative care?   174
- How do I manage mouth problems in palliative care?   175
- How do I manage the psychological care of terminally ill patients?   175

Chapter 10: What else do I need to know?   179

- What are my roles and responsibilities regarding the Mental Health Act?   179
- What issues are involved in obtaining consent?   180
- What are my rights and responsibilities regarding patient records and documentation?   182
- What do I need to know about clinical governance?   184
- What are my rights and responsibilities regarding risk management?   186

References   191

Index   201

Contributors

Claire Agnew
RN(Adult), DipHE Nursing, PGCE, ENB124, ENB 998
Training and Development Sister
Directorate of Medical and A&E Services
University of Leicester Hospitals NHS Trust

Flo Brett
RGN
Clinical Governance Manager
Leicester Royal Infirmary
University Hospitals of Leicester NHS Trust

Nicola Brooks
BSc(Hons), DipHE Nursing, RN, ENB998, ENB931
Practice Development Nurse
Directorate of Surgical Services
Glenfield Hospital
University of Leicester Hospitals NHS Trust

John Fowler
MA, BA, DipN, CertED, RGN, RMN, RCNT, RNT
Principal Lecturer
School of Nursing and Midwifery
De Montfort University
Leicester

Nigel Goodrich
BSc(Hons), DMS, RGN, RMN
Senior Lecturer
School of Nursing and Midwifery
De Montfort University
Leicester

Martyn Geary
MA, BA(Hons), RGN, PGCE(FAHE)
Senior Lecturer – Palliative Care
School of Nursing and Midwifery
De Montfort University
Leicester

Penny Harrison
MA, BSc(Hons), RGN, FETC, CertEd, ENB100
Senior Lecturer – Adult Nursing
School of Nursing and Midwifery
De Montfort University
Leicester

Karen Jackson
BSc(Hons), PG Dip, MMedSci, RGN, RSCN
Clinical Skills Facilitator
Children's Hospital
University Hospitals of Leicester NHS Trust

Annie Law
MA, PGDAdEd, BA(Hons) DPNS, RGN, RNT, ENB100, N59, ENB931, N14
Practitioner/Lecturer
Directorate of Cancer and Haematology
University Hospitals of Leicester HNS Trust
Leicester

Paul Pleasance
EdD, MEd, RGN, ITUCert, PGCE, RNT, ILTM
Principal Lecturer
School of Nursing and Midwifery
De Montfort University
Leicester

Kevin Power
MA, BA(Hons), Dip(N), CertEd, RSCN, RGN
Senior Lecturer
School of Nursing and Midwifery
De Montfort University
Leicester

Paul Rigby
MA, BA(Hons), DipN, DipAdEd, RMN
Senior Lecturer – Mental Health
De Montfort University
Leicester

Wendy Taylor
BSc(Hons), DipHESW, Cert Health Promotion, RGN, ENB931, ENB237, ENB941
Senior Sister
The Leicestershire and Rutland Hospice
Leicester

Keith Todd
RGN, CertEd, ENB199
Senior Lecturer
School of Nursing and Midwifery
De Montfort University
Leicester

Penny Tremayne
MSc, PGDE, BSc(Hons), DipN, RGN
Senior Lecturer – Adult Nursing
School of Nursing and Midwifery
De Montfort University
Leicester

Zoe Wilkes
BSc(Hons), RGN, RSCN
At the time of writing, Senior Nurse
Rainbows Children's Hospice
Loughborough
Leicestershire

Introduction

More than 25 years ago, when I was a junior nurse, one of the most useful books I ever bought was a blank notebook in which I wrote notes and procedures on what to do in certain situations. It is not possible to know how to do everything when you are newly qualified, nor is it possible to carry around a complete set of textbooks for quick reference, hence the idea for this book – a pocket-sized handbook containing ideas, principles and guidelines for a number of common and sometimes unexpected situations that you will probably meet in your first year of practice.

I recently had the privilege of working with a group of clinically based practice development nurses, and discussed with them the possibility of writing such a handbook. They were enthusiastic and wanted to take it on as a project. We collected together all the common situations that a newly qualified staff nurse might face, and then volunteered ourselves, or someone else, to write the answers. The result is this guide: more than 70 questions with answers from 14 different specialists. We aimed to produce an answer for each question that could be read in 5 minutes. This obviously limited the amount of information and rationale that we could include. If you wish to explore any of the subjects in greater depth, you will need to access specialist textbooks. Quay Books is currently producing a complete series of 'Fundamental Aspects of Nursing Practice', which is aimed at the senior student and staff nurse.

This book is intended to be a useful handbook for everyday use – do not leave it on your bookshelf in your room. Keep it on the ward, where you can access it easily. At the end of each chapter there is a blank page for you to add useful local information, such as the telephone number of the infection control nurse, or your own notes on a particular procedure. Add notes to this book and make it your own resource.

I was asked a question recently by a newly qualified nurse – one that does not appear in this book. It was: 'How can I be a really good nurse? My answer was simple: 'Find a really good role model and learn from them.' I hope you want to be a really good nurse: although it is a difficult job, it is one of the most rewarding careers that anyone can have. Work to the best of your ability, work with enthusiasm, listen to your patients and learn from them. Good luck in your nursing career. I hope you find this handbook useful.

Many thanks to all the contributors for their willingness to share their knowledge and experience in the production of this handbook.

John Fowler
De Montfort University
Leicester

Chapter 1

How do I deal with emergencies?

Keith Todd

❖ What do I need to know about cardiorespiratory arrest?
❖ How do I carry out basic life support?
❖ What do I need to know about haemorrhage?
❖ How do I recognise and assess significant haemorrhage?

What do I need to know about cardiorespiratory arrest?

Cardiorespiratory arrest may be a result of a primary airway, breathing or cardiovascular problem (Resuscitation Council (UK), 2002). The cardiovascular and respiratory systems function together to achieve perfusion and oxygenation of body cells, and in this sense are interdependent. Indeed, both systems need to receive a constant supply of oxygenated blood. This interaction and interdependence can have consequences for both systems if either is compromised. For example:

⌘ Hypoxaemia may cause myocardial ischaemia.
⌘ Serious illness, e.g. sepsis, may cause increased oxygen consumption and increased respiratory workload.
⌘ Cardiac failure may be a consequence of respiratory failure, and respiratory failure a consequence of cardiac failure (Resuscitation Council (UK), 2002).

Whenever we talk of a *cardiac* arrest or a *respiratory* arrest, we are referring to a physiological event that ultimately, and occasionally in the very short term, will affect both systems and cause *cardiorespiratory* arrest.

Causes of cardiorespiratory arrest

Jevon (2002) and the Resuscitation Council (UK) (2002) state that cardiac arrest can be caused by a primary airway, respiratory or cardiac problem, or may occur secondary to any life-threatening illness that compromises the airway, breathing or circulation. Both Jevon and the Resuscitation Council categorise the causes of cardiorespiratory arrest under three principal headings:

1. *Airway obstruction, including:*

- Displaced tongue
- Vomit
- Blood

- Foreign body, e.g. foodstuff, a tooth or dentures
- Direct trauma to the face or throat
- Unconsciousness and central nervous system depression, e.g. following head injury, metabolic disorder such as diabetic ketoacidosis or hypoglycaemia, alcohol ingestion, opioid analgesics and general anaesthetics
- Epiglottitis
- Pharyngeal swelling, e.g. caused by infection or oedema
- Laryngospasm
- Bronchospasm or bronchial secretions.

Airway obstruction may be complete or partial, with complete obstruction rapidly leading to cardiac arrest. Partial obstruction often precedes complete obstruction and may also result in cerebral or pulmonary oedema, exhaustion, secondary apnoea and hypoxic brain damage, as well as cardiac arrest (Resuscitation Council (UK), 2002)

2. *Respiratory inadequacy, including:*

⌘ Pulmonary disorders, such as:

- asthma
- pulmonary oedema
- pulmonary embolus
- infection
- aspiration
- exacerbation of chronic obstructive pulmonary disease
- acute respiratory distress syndrome
- haemothorax
- pneumothorax or tension pneumothorax.

⌘ Reduced or abolished respiratory drive as a result of the factors that cause central nervous system depression (see above).

⌘ Reduced respiratory effort caused by muscle weakness or nerve damage associated with conditions such as:

- myasthenia gravis
- Guillain-Barré syndrome
- multiple sclerosis
- poliomyelitis
- motor neurone disease
- muscular dystrophy.

3. *Cardiac abnormalities*
These may be further classified as *primary* or *secondary* cardiac abnormalities (Resuscitation Council (UK), 2002).

Primary abnormalities that may cause cardiac arrest include:

- myocardial ischaemia and infarction
- hypertensive heart disease
- valve disease
- drugs such as tricyclic antidepressants, digoxin and anti-arrhythmic drugs
- acidosis
- electrolyte imbalance
- hypothermia
- electrocution.

Secondary abnormalities that may cause cardiac arrest include:
- asphyxia due to airway obstruction or apnoea
- tension pneumothorax
- acute blood loss
- severe hypoxaemia
- septic shock.

Causes of isolated respiratory arrest

Moulton and Yates (1999) identify four main circumstances in which isolated respiratory arrest, or failure of ventilation in the presence of a clear airway and a central pulse, may occur:

- Poisoning with narcotic agents
- General brainstem depression associated with, for example, trauma, stroke or drugs
- Respiratory failure
- Neuromuscular paralysis.

The Resuscitation Council (UK) (2002) state that respiratory arrest often results from a combination of factors; for example, a chest infection, muscle weakness or fractured ribs will compound the situation in a patient who already has chronic respiratory inadequacy, leading to exhaustion, which further depresses respiratory function. As described above, severe respiratory inadequacy will ultimately lead to cardiac arrest.

How do I handle the situation?

Ultimately, whether the patient suffers an isolated respiratory arrest initially or a cardiorespiratory arrest immediately, the emergency response follows guidelines established by the Resuscitation Council (UK) (2002, 2000a). The Council acknowledges that the level of resuscitation skills required by individual members of the healthcare team will differ according to their role in the service. This applies equally to in-hospital healthcare staff (Resuscitation Council (UK), 2000b) as well as those in primary care (Resuscitation Council (UK), 2001).

Within hospital practice, the Resuscitation Council (UK) (2000b) recommends that all doctors, nursing staff and allied health professionals (e.g. physiotherapists, radiographers and occupational therapists) should have basic life support (BLS) training. This would include airway adjuncts if immediately available. Nursing staff should have been trained to a standard and level of competence compatible with their level of experience and expected duties within the hospital. Ideally, within specialist areas, appropriate nursing staff should hold a valid Resuscitation Council (UK) Advanced Life Support (ALS) Certificate.

Within primary care, the Resuscitation Council (UK) (2001) recommends that all those in direct contact with patients should be trained in BLS using an airway adjunct, such as a pocket mask, and related resuscitation skills, such as the recovery position. Doctors, nurses and other paramedical workers, such as physiotherapists, should also be trained to use an automated external defibrillator effectively.

Within the primary care setting, however, community nursing staff may find themselves as a first responder, on their own with a collapsed patient who may have a respiratory or cardiorespiratory arrest within the home. In this situation they may have to call for paramedic support and undertake BLS until they arrive with ALS equipment and expertise on board.

Emphasis continues to be placed on the rapid initiation of BLS as an immediate first responder intervention, until ALS equipment and staff arrive on the scene.

How do I carry out basic life support?

Sequence of interventions for adult BLS (Resuscitation Council (UK), 2002)

Practice points about this sequence of actions, focusing on the use of airway adjuncts and in-hospital BLS, are provided within the sequence.

Assessing patient responsiveness:

- Ensure that the location around you is safe for both you and the patient.
- Gently but firmly *shake* the patient's shoulders and enquire *loudly*, 'Are you all right?'
- If there is no response to this, *shout for help*.

Assessing the airway:

- If you cannot assess the patient fully in the position he is found in, carefully turn him on his back.
- If there is no suspicion of cervical spine injury suggested by the incident, or from any available history from a witness, open the airway using a *head-tilt, chin-lift* maneouvre.
- Place a hand on the patient's forehead and gently tilt the head backwards,

keeping thumb and forefinger free to close the nose if rescue breathing needs to be provided.
- Perform a visual check of the airway and a manual (or suction) removal of any foreign body and/or debris. If suction is used to clear any blood, saliva, foodstuff or gastric contents from the upper airway, this should be performed with a rigid, wide-bore catheter, such as a Yankauer sucker.
- At the same time, using *one or two fingers* on the *bony point of the chin only*, lift the chin to open the airway.
- You may have to loosen any tight clothing around the neck. Dentures may be left in situ if they are firmly in place; they help to maintain the shape and structure of the mouth and may make it easier to create and maintain an airtight seal around it. *They should be removed if loose*, as they may become a risk to the airway.

> **Practice points about this sequence of actions**
> - Use the chin lift rather than a hand placed underneath the patient's neck. The anatomy of the mouth, tongue and oropharynx means that this achieves a more patent airway and less resistance to airflow, and hence easier assessment of breathing and subsequent assisted respiration, if required.
> - Use one or two fingers only on the chin. Using the entire hand on and under the chin tends to impinge on the floor of the mouth and press these soft tissues up into the oropharynx, occluding the airway.

Assessing breathing:

- Keeping the airway open, *look, listen and feel for 10 seconds* before deciding that breathing is absent. This requires you to:
  - *look* for chest movements (much easier to ascertain if you align yourself parallel with the front of the patient's chest, looking down along the anterior chest wall)
  - *listen* for breath sounds from the patient's mouth
  - *feel* for air upon your own cheek.

All three of these observations should take place in the same 10 seconds.

> **Practice point about this sequence of actions**
> - Appropriately trained and competent staff should be able to assess circulation by checking for the presence or absence of the carotid pulse at the same time as checking for breathing.

If the patient is breathing normally:

- Turn him into the recovery position.
- Summon help or go for help if you are on your own.
- Check for continued breathing on your return.

If the patient is not breathing:

- Send for help, if no-one has arrived already in response to your first shout, or go to summon help if you are on your own.
- On your return, if you haven't already done so, carefully turn the patient onto his back.
- Provide two *effective* rescue breaths initially (each must make the chest rise and fall):

  - Maintain the *head-tilt, chin-lift* position while ventilating the patient.
  - Pinch the soft part of the nose and place your lips around the mouth. Do not forget the need to obtain a good seal around the patient's mouth and to provide *two, even, controlled* rescuer breaths.
  - Only a small amount of resistance should be felt during mouth-to-mouth ventilation, and each inflation *should take around 2 seconds.*

Practice points about this sequence of actions

- The amount of air required in an adult is around 700–1000ml (Resuscitation Council (UK), 2000a), or, expressed slightly differently, 10ml/kg (Resuscitation Council (UK), 2002). This is, of course, difficult to estimate during basic life support, and in practice is the amount required to produce a visible lifting of the chest.

- Remember the potential dangers of over-inflation (gastric dilatation and regurgitation and aspiration of stomach contents).

- The Resuscitation Council (UK) (2002) states that the exact timing is not critical: wait for the chest to fall completely, usually taking 2–4 seconds, and then give another inflation.

- If in-hospital airway management and ventilation are required, this should be undertaken with the most appropriate equipment immediately available.
  - Simple adjuncts such as a pocket mask, which can be used in conjunction with an oral airway, ought to be readily available in a hospital setting.
  - Alternatively, a laryngeal mask airway and bag-valve apparatus, or bag-valve-mask device, can be used.
  - Supplemental oxygen should be given as soon as possible (Resuscitation Council (UK), 2002). When this is given with an unprotected airway (essentially without tracheal intubation in situ), a lower tidal volume of 400–600 ml should be used.

How do I deal with emergencies?

If any difficulty is experienced while attempting to inflate the patient's chest:

- Try to tilt the head further and increase chin lift.
- Recheck that the mouth is clear of any obstruction. Removal of an obstruction, once again, can be achieved by a careful sweep of the mouth with an index finger or by suction, if available.
- Ensure that your lips are well sealed around the patient's mouth.
- Make up to *five* attempts to achieve *two effective* rescuer breaths.
- Even if these are unsuccessful, move on to assess the patient's circulation.

Assessing the circulation:

- Look for any signs of movement, including swallowing or breathing (more than the occasional gasp).

- If you have been trained to do it, *check the carotid pulse*. Check for a *maximum of 10 seconds*.

- If you are confident that you can detect signs of a circulation:

  - Continue to provide rescue breathing until the patient starts to breathe on his own.
  - About every 10 breaths (or about every minute), recheck for any signs of a circulation, checking for a maximum of 10 seconds each time.
  - If the patient starts to breathe normally on his own but remains unconscious, turn him into the recovery position. You should stay with the patient and be ready to turn him on to his back once more and restart rescue breathing if he stops breathing again.

- If there is no pulse or other sign of a circulation, or you are at all unsure, start chest compressions.

- Locate correct position on the chest. This can be found by using the hand nearest the patient's feet to locate the lower half of the sternum:

  - Use your index and middle fingers to identify the lower rib border on the side of the abdomen nearest you.
  - Keep your fingers together and run them up the edge of this border to the point where the ribs meet the sternum.
  - With your middle finger on this point, place your index finger on the sternum.
  - Slide the heel of your other hand down the centre of the sternum until it reaches your index finger. This should be in the middle of the lower half of the sternum, directly overlying the patient's heart.
  - Put the heel of your other hand on top of the first hand.
  - Fingers can be extended or interlocked and lifted to avoid putting

pressure over the patient's ribs. This avoids dissipating compression forces and potentially also breaking the patient's ribs.
- Likewise, do not put pressure over the upper abdomen or xiphisternum.

⌘ Start chest compressions:

- Position yourself directly above the patient's chest, with your arms straight, and press down on the sternum to depress it between 4 and 5 cm.
- Release the pressure without allowing your hand to lose contact with the patient's chest, and repeat this at a rate of around 100 times a minute, completing 15 compressions per cycle. Allow equal time for the compression phase and the release phase, to allow the chest to return to its normal position after each one.

⌘ Combine rescue breathing with compressions:

- After each cycle of 15 compressions, tilt the head and lift the chin again and give another two rescue breaths. In-hospital resuscitation with simple adjuncts may involve the use of the bag-valve-mask or laryngeal mask airway and bag-valve device.
- Relocate the correct hand position on the chest and repeat the 15 compressions phase, continuing this cycle of compressions and breaths in a 15:2 ratio.

Practice points about this sequence of actions
Ensure:

❖ **Correct hand position throughout the procedure**
- Keeping your hands in contact with the chest throughout each phase of compressions will promote this.
- Relocating the correct position, if you are performing both rescuer breathing and compressions, can be achieved without hurrying by following the above advice. With practice you will become more fluent at this manoeuvre.
- On collapsed patients with peripheral pooling of blood during an arrest, you can often see an imprint of your previous hand position, providing a general guide to location as you return to the compression phase.

❖ **Correct body posture**
Performing compressions in clinical practice can be quite tiring. Keeping your arms straight, pivoting at the hip and using your upper body weight is less tiring than trying to apply pressure using your arm muscles. Pressure should be firm, controlled, and applied vertically.

❖ **Correct depth of compression (4–5cm in an adult patient)**
This is difficult to estimate from a correct body posture, i.e. vertically above the patient's chest. In most cases, you will encounter a certain resistance as you approach the natural limits to the patient's chest wall 'elasticity'.

Practice points about this sequence of actions (cont'd)

- **Correct compression rate (about 100/min)**
  Counting aloud '1 and 2 and …12 and 13–14–15' helps you to get into a rhythm and also provides any second person providing inflations with an audible cue.
- **Equal compression/relaxation phases**
  Patients' chests often do not rebound as readily as a training manikin! You need to allow the ventricles to refill adequately to maintain optimum cardiac output with your compressions.
- **Correct ratio of compression:ventilation (15:2)**
  This allows a more fluent resuscitation event than the previous 5:1 ratio, enhancing coronary and cerebral perfusion pressures during compressions. The greater the number of compressions, the greater the benefit, even in the face of fewer ventilations (Kern *et al*, 1998)
- Finally, remember that even competent, well-performed cardiac compressions will only achieve a cardiac output that is, at best, *less than 30% of normal* (Resuscitation Council (UK), 2002).
- *Any deviation from good technique detracts from this, and further compromises the patient unnecessarily.*

The Resuscitation Council (UK) (2002) recommends that, as the likelihood of BLS alone restoring effective cardiac activity is remote, time should not be wasted in further checks for the return of a pulse.

If the patient makes any sort of movement or takes a spontaneous breath, check the carotid pulse, taking no more than 10 seconds to do this. **Otherwise do not interrupt CPR.**

Continue resuscitation until:

- Qualified help, such as a medical emergency team with ALS skills and equipment, arrives and takes over.
- The patient shows signs of life.
- You become exhausted.

A final note

The sections on cardiorespiratory arrest and BLS provide an overview of your actions, essentially as a first responder in either primary or secondary care, and summarise a great deal of information and guidance available from the Resuscitation Council (UK) and other authors in the field.

These guidelines are under constant review. Modifications are made to individual actions within the sequence and to the actual sequence of interventions itself as new evidence comes to light. It is essential that you keep yourself up to date with these (see www.resus.org.uk for information).

Theoretical instruction and aide-mémoires such as this are no substitute for approved education and training in the skills, together with an integral assessment of competence required to practise these safely. You may find that the resuscitation training department within your own healthcare trust takes the same view, and will seek you out, on your appointment and regularly thereafter, to keep you up to date.

The Resuscitation Council (UK) guidelines have removed the confusion and occasional fear previously associated with the management of cardiorespiratory arrest. If you have the opportunity subsequently to participate in the team management of one of these events, there is no better place to be than right in the centre, performing chest compressions. If you demonstrate competent and effective skills in this, no-one will bother you, other than occasionally to ask if you would like a rest. You will rarely find yourself in such an absorbing, interactive learning situation.

What do I need to know about haemorrhage?

Haemorrhage (*Box 1.1*) – the loss of whole blood from the intravascular compartment – is the commonest cause of hypovolaemia (Collins, 2000) or hypovolaemic shock (Rice, 1991). The loss of intravascular blood volume decreases the venous return to the heart, leading to a reduction in cardiac output. This results in poor perfusion of the tissues and cells, which in turn causes widespread disruption to cellular metabolism. Shock, whatever the initial cause and underlying pathophysiology, is defined as a potentially life-threatening failure of the cardiovascular system to perfuse body tissues adequately (Edwards, 2001, Hand, 2001). Inadequate tissue perfusion results in a lack of cellular oxygen and widespread disruption of cellular metabolism (Cohen, 2003). If this is not reversed, cell death occurs, affecting tissues and organs within the body, leading ultimately to multi-organ failure and potentially death of the individual.

Box 1.1
Causes of significant haemorrhage (Wyatt et al, 1999)

Upper gastrointestinal bleeding
- Peptic ulceration
- Oesophagitis
- Gastritis
- Oesophageal varices
- Mallory–Weiss tear
- Gastric carcinoma

Obstetric conditions
- Ruptured ectopic pregnancy
- Placenta praevia
- Abruption of placenta

Lower gastrointestinal bleeding
(20% of acute gastrointestinal bleeding is from the colon or rectum)
- Commonest causes are angiodysplasia and bleeding from diverticulae

Trauma
- Musculoskeletal
- Intra-abdominal
- Intrathoracic
- Pelvic

How do I deal with emergencies?

The classification of shock is variously described as comprising either five (Collins, 2000; Edwards, 2001; Jones, 2003) or three different types (Rice, 1991; Hand, 2001; O'Reilly, 2003). These are essentially based on the underlying condition and associated pathophysiology (see *Box 1.2* for summary).

Box 1.2
Two different classifications of types of shock

First classification	Second classification
Hypovolaemic shock	Hypovolaemic shock
Cardiogenic chock	Cardiogenic shock
Anaphylactic shock	Distributive (or vasogenic) shock incorporating:
Neurogenic shock	• anaphylactic shock
	• neurogenic shock
Septic shock	• septic shock

What happens during hypovolaemic (haemorrhagic) shock?

In hypovolaemic (haemorrhagic) shock, there are broadly accepted 'stages' of shock, which are linked to the body's physiological response to the volume of blood loss. Some authors describe three stages (Edwards, 2001; Hand, 2001), while others describe a fourth – the 'initial' stage (Collins, 2000). Each stage is broadly associated with a range of clinical signs and symptoms incorporating patient's appearance, level of consciousness and vital signs parameters.

Compensatory (compensated) stage

This early stage reflects the initiation of the body's normal homeostatic mechanism to maintain cardiovascular stability in the face of blood loss through haemorrhage. It a consequence of a sympathetic response, via the autonomic nervous system, to stimuli received from aortic and carotid baroreceptors and chemoreceptors, which results in the release of adrenaline and noradrenaline. Adrenaline increases arteriolar resistance and has a chronotropic effect, which increases the heart rate, and an inotropic effect, which increases myocardial contractility. All of these effects help to maintain the blood pressure in the event of falling cardiac output resulting from a reduction in blood volume. Noradrenaline is released more slowly than adrenaline, and results in intense vasoconstriction, reducing the potential venous blood volume contained within the systemic veins during the non-shock state, contributing to venous return and consequently to cardiac output to maintain blood pressure.

Reduced renal blood flow also results in activation of the renin-angiotensin system. As well as having a vasoconstrictor effect, angiotensin II also stimulates the secretion of aldosterone, which causes the retention of sodium and water.

As a consequence of the rising serum sodium level, osmoreceptors in the hypothalamus stimulate the release of antidiuretic hormone. The end result of these two mechanisms is the retention of sodium and water, a rise in blood pressure due to increased blood volume and vasoconstriction, and a reduction in urine output.

If the patient is treated in the early compensatory stage of hypovolaemic shock, the prognosis has been described as excellent (Edwards, 2001); however, if the hypovolaemic shock progresses to the next stage – progressive or uncompensated shock – the prognosis is less predictable.

Progressive (uncompensated) stage

If blood loss is not corrected, ultimately arterial blood pressure falls, resulting in widespread cellular hypoxia and dysfunction within body tissues and organs (Edwards, 2001; Hand, 2001).

Refractory stage

Continuing cellular and organ dysfunction leads to an irreversible deterioration in the patient's condition. At this stage it may be possible to raise the arterial pressure to within relatively normal limits, but the associated cellular disruption continues and death is inevitable (Collins, 2000; Edwards, 2001).

How do I recognise and assess significant haemorrhage?

In hypovolaemic shock, as with any other type of shock, the role of the nurse is to recognise, assess, monitor and treat the condition.

Recognition of an obvious or potential haemorrhage will depend on the patient's immediate presentation and associated history, together with any recent medical or healthcare history, if this is available.

Signs and symptoms observable in the patient will generally follow a broad pattern depending on what stage of blood loss and shock the patient presents in. The American College of Surgeons (ACS) (1989) classification of the degree of haemorrhage has been broadly adopted in the UK. The blood volume loss ranges from class 1 to class 4, each class representing an increasing loss as a percentage range of total blood volume. Each subsequent class is again broadly associated with a deterioration in the parameters of a number of signs and symptoms, allowing the nurse to assess and monitor the patient's status.

Occasionally, the percentage of blood volume loss allied to each 'class' in some of the UK literature is slightly different. Although the classes reflect a pattern of clinical features, it is important to acknowledge that individual patients may vary in their presentation, and also that we ought to be aware of trends, as well as absolute values.

Table 1.1 details the signs and symptoms associated with classes 1–4 haemorrhage.

Table 1.1 Signs and symptoms seen in classes 1–4 haemorrhage (ACS, 1989)

Class 1 haemorrhage 0–15% blood volume loss (≤750 ml) Initial homeostatic response	Class 2 haemorrhage 15–30% blood volume loss (750–1500 ml) Compensatory stage Sympathetic stimulation	Class 3 haemorrhage 30–40% blood volume loss (1500–2000 ml) Progressive stage Decreasing tissue perfusion	Class 4 haemorrhage >40% blood volume loss (>2000 ml) Refractory (irreversible) stage Vital organ failure
Signs and symptoms	**Signs and symptoms**	**Signs and symptoms**	**Signs and symptoms**
Normal heart rate	Tachycardia (>100 beats/min)	Heart rate >120 beats/min, thready pulse	Heart rate >140 beats/min, thready pulse. May have a bradycardia (preterminal event)
Normal blood pressure (BP)	Normal/slightly reduced BP	Marked hypotension: systolic BP 80–90 mmHg	Pulse pressure further reduced (perhaps no diastolic)
Normal/widened pulse pressure: (systolic:diastolic: pulse pressure ratio 3:2:1)	Pulse pressure narrowed: (minimal systolic change/raised diastolic value – indicates significant blood loss)	Pulse pressure further narrowed. Systolic and diastolic both reducing	
Respiratory rate: normal (10–20 minutes)	Raised respiratory rate	Respiratory rate 30–40/min	Respirations >35/min
Normal capillary refill (≤2 s)	Delayed capillary refill (>2s)	Poor capillary refill	Skin cold, mottled, cyanotic deoxygenated blood pooling in periphery. Marked diaphoresis
Pale pink, cool skin	Slightly pale, cool skin	Pale, cold moist skin	
Normal urine output (≥30 ml/h)	Reduced urine output (20–30 ml/h)	Reduced urine output (5–15 ml/h)	Oliguria/anuria
Slightly anxious	Mildly apprehensive, oriented	Anxious, confused	Confused or lethargic. Conscious level further reduced. May be unconscious after 50% blood loss

See also 'Notes on Table 1.1' on p.14

Notes on Table 1.1

- Volumes of blood loss given are for the average 70 kg man (ACS, 1989).

- Pulse pressure is the difference between the systolic and diastolic readings. Normal systolic:diastolic:pulse pressure ratio is approximately 3:2:1 (e.g. a patient with a 'normal' blood pressure of 120/80 mmHg would have a pulse pressure of 40 mmHg).

- Capillary refill time should be measured by raising the patient's hand or foot above the level of the heart, pressing gently on a peripheral area, such as a nail bed, for 5 seconds to blanch the area before releasing, and measuring the time taken for it to re-perfuse and regain its normal colour. Normal capillary refill time in an ambient temperature environment would be up to 2 seconds.

How can I estimate blood pressure during blood loss?

Blood pressure can be difficult to measure in the face of continuing haemorrhage. You can try to palpate the systolic blood pressure by inflating the sphygmomanometer cuff on the patient's arm until you obliterate the brachial or radial pulse. The cuff can then be slowly released until you feel the brachial or radial pulse. The systolic blood pressure should be recorded as the mmHg value corresponding to the first pulsation (McCormac, 1990).

There are other 'rule of thumb' methods of estimating systolic blood pressure (McCormac, 1990):

- If you can palpate a radial pulse the systolic blood pressure is probably at least 80 mmHg.

- If you can feel a femoral pulse the systolic blood pressure is probably at least 70 mmHg.

- If you can feel a carotid pulse the systolic blood pressure is probably at least 60 mmHg.

These indicators are also incorporated within the ACS (1989) Advanced Trauma Life Support guidelines. However, these indicators have recently been challenged by Deakin and Low (2000), who found that they can be inaccurate and generally overestimate the patient's systolic blood pressure, and hence underestimate the degree of blood loss and subsequent hypovolaemia.

Because of the body's homeostatic response to blood loss, measuring blood pressure in the compensatory stage is not always a reliable indicator of the patient's actual status, and emphasis should be placed on observations, such as the patient's skin perfusion, respiratory rate, temperature on touch, pulse rate and general condition (Hand, 2001; Kolecki, 2001). In an otherwise healthy adult with ongoing haemorrhage, hypotension may not become evident until as much as 30% of blood volume has been lost (Kolecki, 2001; Cohen, 2003). Patients who are taking beta-blockers may also not present with a tachycardia, whatever their degree of blood loss (Kolecki, 2001). Again, you should be looking at the overall trend when monitoring the patient's signs and symptoms.

How do I treat significant haemorrhage?

The immediate management of a patient's haemorrhage will depend upon its presentation: the care of a patient who presents with an epistaxis will obviously differ from that of a road traffic accident victim who is brought to the emergency department, in terms of the degree and number of nursing and medical interventions.

We should not underestimate the psychological impact of trauma or blood loss for the patient, even those presenting with a relatively small bleed. Patient safety, comfort and reassurance should be acknowledged and preserved throughout nursing and medical interventions. All patients, including those who self-refer with a relatively small haemorrhage, should be allowed to sit or lie down as appropriate, and also need to be kept informed, reassured and supported throughout their immediate care. These principles apply equally to those who present with more significant haemorrhage.

The immediate goals in the management of hypovolaemic shock are set out in *Box 1.3* (Hand, 2001; Kolecki, 2001.

Box 1.3
Immediate management of hypovolaemic shock

- Maximise ventilation and oxygenation in the patient.
- Fluid resuscitation: optimise intravascular volume by appropriate, rapid intravenous infusion.
- Locate and correct the underlying cause of the haemorrhage.

Ventilation and oxygen delivery

The patient's airway should be immediately assessed and secured following current immediate life support guidelines (Resuscitation Council (UK), 2002).

If the patient is not responsive, this may include:

- Positioning the airway, using a head-tilt, chin-lift manoeuvre.
- A jaw thrust technique if there is any likelihood or history of head or cervical spine injury.
- A check to see if the patient is breathing.

If airway management and ventilation are required, this should be undertaken with the most appropriate equipment immediately available.

- Simple adjuncts such as a pocket mask, which can be used in conjunction with an oral airway, ought to be readily available in a hospital setting.

- Alternatively, a laryngeal mask airway and bag-valve apparatus, or bag-valve-mask device can be used.

- High-flow supplemental oxygen should be administered to all potentially shocked patients as soon as possible (Kolecki, 2001).

Fluid resuscitation

Resuscitation should be undertaken with warmed intravenous (IV) fluids. Two large-bore IV lines should be inserted immediately to enable simultaneous administration of blood and fluids (Hand, 2001). These should be 16 gauge or larger. Fluid flow through a cannula is inversely proportional to its length and directly proportional to its internal diameter. Short large-bore cannulae are therefore ideal (Kolecki, 2001), a large calibre being more significant than the length.

Preferential sites for IV cannulae, in order of priority are:

1. Percutaneous peripheral access through the forearm or antecubital veins. (This avoids potential leakage of IV replacement fluids immediately into the abdominal or pelvic cavities following trauma in these regions.)
2. Cutdown of the saphenous vein or arm veins.
3. Central venous access.

Nursing staff should anticipate these interventions and prepare for and initiate peripheral IV access (according to local policy) or prepare for and assist with cutdown and central line placement by medical staff.

Which IV fluid?

There has been a great deal of controversy regarding the IV fluid of choice (principally colloids *versus* crystalloids) for fluid resuscitation (Cohen, 2003). Despite many studies, neither fluid has demonstrated a difference in patient outcome. Current recommendations still advocate the use of normal saline or lactated Ringer solution (Kolecki, 2001).

Initial fluid resuscitation is performed with a warmed isotonic crystalloid such as lactated Ringer solution or normal saline (Hand, 2001; Kolecki, 2001).

- Where significant haemorrhage is a likely factor in the presentation and fluid has been commenced, an initial bolus of 1–2 litres will be given to an adult and a bolus of 20 ml/kg to a paediatric patient. In either case, the patient's response to this will be assessed to determine further interventions.

⌘ If the patient's vital signs return to normal, the patient may be monitored to ensure ongoing stability. A small group of patients will remain stable following the initial fluid bolus. Such patients will generally have lost less than 20% of their blood volume. Blood may be taken at this point to be sent for typing and crossmatching (ACS, 1989; Kolecki, 2001).

⌘ The largest group of patients will respond transiently to this initial fluid bolus. Crystalloid infusion should continue and type-specific blood obtained.

⌘ If there is little or no improvement or if, as IV fluids are slowed, vital signs deteriorate once again, crystalloid infusion should continue and type O blood given (Kolecki, 2001). Many of these patients will have lost 20–40% of their blood volume, or will still be bleeding (ACS, 1989). This group reqires urgent surgical assessment.

⌘ Type O, Rh-negative blood should be given to females within the child-bearing age range to avoid sensitization and future complications during childbirth (Kolecki, 2001).

⌘ If a patient presents in a moribund state, towards the class 4 haemorrhage end of the spectrum, both crystalloid fluids and type O blood should be given from the outset. Again, urgent surgical assessment and/or intervention is required here.

⌘ The patient's position can be altered to improve venous return and cardiac output and hence aid perfusion of vital organs. Lowering the head of the patient's trolley or bed will help to achieve this, and increase blood flow to the brain (Kolecki, 2001).

Locating and correcting the underlying cause of the haemorrhage

This will depend on the site of the haemorrhage. Bleeding from the head, ears, eyes, nose and throat are usually obvious (Bozeman, 2001). These may be reported by the patient or be clearly visible to the assessing nurse. The scalp has the most richly perfused cutaneous blood supply in the body (Ellis, 1997) and can produce a significant haemorrhage (Bozeman, 2001).

Surface haemorrhage from other areas may not be so immediately apparent and will probably require exposure of the patient.

⌘ Overt bleeding to the body surface can be controlled with direct pressure over the site.

⌘ Care should be taken over the site of a suspected fracture. Excessive pressure here may cause further displacement of bone ends, associated muscle injury and damage, and further bleeding. Kolecki (2001) advocates the use of traction with long bone fractures to reduce blood loss from the fracture site. See *Box 1.4* for potential blood loss from fracture sites (Collins, 2000).

✣ Upper and lower limbs may be elevated on pillows, in conjunction with direct pressure if appropriate, to reduce blood loss from distal sites.

Box 1.4 Estimated blood loss from fracture sites	
Pelvis	3000 ml
Femur	1000 ml
Tibia	650 ml

Associated nursing practice

✣ Catheterisation will normally be performed to allow accurate monitoring and recording of fluid balance during fluid resuscitation in significant shock states. Nurses should anticipate and prepare for this procedure.

✣ Observation of vital signs, and monitoring and documenting the parameters in *Table 1.1,* should also be performed throughout this phase. Neurological status should be monitored using a recognised tool, such as the Glasgow Coma Scale (Hand, 2001), which assesses and measures the patient's eye-opening response, and best motor and verbal responses. Communication of these observations and associated trends in values should be communicated immediately to other members of the attending team.

✣ Complications of fluid resuscitation can occur, and observation of the patient throughout the immediate fluid resuscitation phase is vital (Hand, 2001). The risk of these complications is increased in older patients and those with pre-existing cardiovascular disease.

✣ In addition to the parameters in *Table 1.1*, the patient's temperature should be monitored to check for infusion-induced hypothermia (Hand, 2001), which is perhaps more likely to occur if fluid-warming devices are not immediately available. The patient's jugular vein should also be observed for signs of distension, indicating fluid overload (Hand, 2001).

Final point

Uncontrolled, untreated blood loss will inevitably lead to hypovolaemic shock. Such an event is a medical emergency, and nurses must be able to identify and treat patients in shock. As Collins (2000) states:

> *'Regular assessment and accurate monitoring of patients most at risk of shock is crucial and the nurse must ensure these skills are incorporated into his or her daily practice.'*

How do I deal with emergencies?

Personal notes and contacts

Chapter 2

How do I deal with the unexpected?

Kevin Power

- How do I deal with difficult questions?
- How do I deal with complaints?
- How do I deal with aggressive patients or relatives?
- What is involved in incident reporting?
- What are my responsibilities in reporting malpractice?
- What can I do about bullying within the organization?
- What do I do if a patient wants to self-discharge?
- How do I deal with MRSA?

How do I deal with difficult questions?

Difficult questions probably fall into two categories: those to which you do not know the answer and those that you are not sure how to answer.

The first type of difficult question is probably relatively easy to deal with. Being honest and telling the questioner that you do not know the answer is the best response. Trying to bluff an answer is fraught with difficulty, as it is always likely that you will be caught out. Many newly qualified staff nurses perceive that other people expect them to 'know everything' because they are qualified, regardless of the length of their experience (Lathlean, 1987; Shand, 1987; Power, 1996; Charnley, 1999). However, it is unreasonable to expect anyone to know the answer to all the questions that may be asked. There should be no shame in admitting that you are temporarily at a loss for an answer. Obviously you will promise to find out the answer or find someone who can give that answer, and it is important to keep that promise.

The second type of difficult question is altogether more challenging. This type of question may fall into one of two categories. The answer to the question may be rather complex and the difficulty here is making sure that your explanation is easily understood by the questioner. The best way to approach such situations is to build up a personal 'thesaurus' of everyday words that mean the same as or explain technical jargon. For example, a patient may ask what a lesion is as the doctor mentioned this to them. This word can have a variety of meanings, ranging from an innocent wart to a potentially devastating cancer. Having a ready response that can explain such words in lay terms will enable you to ensure that patients or relatives understand their care and treatment (see *Case Study 2.1*).

The second category of question that you may not be sure how to answer is probably those that have an ethical component. An example of this would be

> **Case study 2.1**
>
> **Amit Shah** had recently been diagnosed as having leukaemia. He said to the nurse caring for him that the doctor had explained the disease to him but he did not really understand what the doctor was saying as he had used some long unintelligible words. The nurse asked some basic questions of Amit in order to establish how much he did know. She then gathered pens and paper and drew a picture using an analogy of opposing armies fighting a battle to explain how the disease happened and progressed. The combination of the use of lay language and pictures enabled Amit to understand much clearer what was going on in his body.

when a patient asks what is wrong with him, when you know a decision has been made by the multidisciplinary team not to reveal the true diagnosis at this point in the patient's care. The *Code of Professional Conduct* (Nursing & Midwifery Council [NMC], 2004a) states, in clause 3.1:

> *'All patients and clients have a right to receive information about their condition ... Information should be accurate, truthful and presented in such a way as to make it easily understood.'*

Some have argued that physicians (and by extension any health professional) should '...cultivate lying as a fine art' (Collins, 1988) in order to bolster the hopes of the patient, who may be seriously ill, and prevent them from losing the will to live. Whether everyone could learn to lie effectively and control their facial expression is a moot point. Jackson (2001) is unequivocal in her condemnation of all lie, whether trivial or serious. I always advise my students to avoid all lies in their practice. Anything that has the potential to reduce a patient's or relative's trust in nurses should probably be avoided; lying is fairly certain to reduce that trust and all lies have the potential to be discovered (see *Case Study 2.2*).

> **Case study 2.2**
>
> **Sally Dent,** the mother of 5-year-old Ben, insisted that nurses did not tell her son that he would have any pain following some relatively minor surgery. No amount of persuasion would shift Sally and she remained insistent. The nurses decided that they would accede to Sally's wish as they reasoned she knew her son best. Ben did ask 'Will it hurt?', and the nurse kept silent when his mum assured him that it would not hurt.
>
> After returning from theatre, Ben, despite having received analgesia as part of the anaesthetic, was in some discomfort although not significant pain. He became very distressed, shouting at the nurses that they had lied to him as it did hurt. The rest of his short stay in hospital was difficult as he was unwilling for the nurses to do much for him.

Generally, if a person asks a question it is because they want to hear the answer. When a patient has a serious condition with a poor prognosis, many staff nurses tell me that they have the feeling the patient already knows and is merely seeking confirmation. Thus the honest and truthful answer may not be a shock to the patient. That does not mean that the patient will not become upset, and you must prepare yourself to provide appropriate comfort in such situations. There is, of course, a potential risk of upsetting other members of the team by revealing the truth after a decision has been made to withhold a diagnosis. A professional judgment has to be made whether to reveal the truth or not.

There are also ways of addressing such questions without the need to resort to lying. One could truthfully answer: 'I am afraid I cannot answer that question at the moment'. This does run the risk of the patient then saying: 'Why, because you don't know or because you don't want to tell me?' A reasonable response could then be that you are not the best person to ask and that you will arrange for them to speak to someone who can answer their questions effectively.

How do I deal with complaints?

In his report for 2001–2002, the Health Service Ombudsman stated that complaints about care are often aggravated by sometimes simple failures to apply the complaints procedures properly (Health Service Ombudsman, 2002). The problem with some complaints is that they may begin as minor issues, but, if not dealt with properly, can become a major confrontation. Of the 281 complaints upheld by the Health Service Ombudsman in 2001–2, 78 were about the handling of complaints. The way a nurse deals with a complaint at the very beginning of the process can thus have an effect on the whole course of that complaint.

The simplest way to deal with complaints is to prevent them occurring in the first place. Be on the lookout for signs that a patient or relative is getting irritated; don't wait for the complaint – ask whether there is a problem. I remember sitting completing a duty rota and overhearing a father sounding cross on the telephone outside the ward office. It was clear that something was wrong. When I went to investigate, it seems that no-one had told him what was going on with his young daughter, who had been admitted as an emergency, and he had an important business meeting to attend. When I asked the staff caring for the child to explain what the delay was and the likely time frame for her admission, he was able to make some arrangements with his work and became much calmer.

If this situation had been ignored it is highly likely that a formal complaint would have been lodged. However, it is unlikely that the health service is going to please all of the people all of the time, no matter how high your personal standards of care or how good your communication skills. Patients and relatives may be in pain or anxious and certainly in a strange environment. Additionally, as staff are under pressure because of high workloads and staff shortages, there are always likely to be complaints of some kind or another.

Most NHS trusts actively seek feedback from patients and service users as part of clinical governance (Robotham, 2001). This may enable trusts to forestall complaints through improvements to the service. It may also encourage more people to complain. Each trust will have protocols and policies in place for dealing with formal complaints and you should be familiar with these. Let us focus for the purposes of this section on those situations where a relative or patient makes a verbal complaint to you.

Consider the following:

Think of a time when you have complained about something:

- What was the cause of the complaint?
- Who did you complain to?
- How was the complaint dealt with?
- How did this make you feel?

Most complaints are fairly mundane, but no matter how trivial to the member of staff, all are important to the complainant. When thinking about times when I have complained, the response of the person I have complained to has had a great impact on how far I wanted to take the complaint and the level of redress I expected. So how do you, as the nurse receiving a verbal complaint, respond? The Wilson Report (Department of Health, 1994) identified several lessons from the private sector:

- *Complainants do want an apology, even if the organisation was not at fault*

    This does not mean accepting responsibility for the problem. Just saying sorry that the person feels there is a problem may at least show that you are acknowledging their concerns.

- *Complainants want a speedy response*

    Show that you are willing to take action immediately, even if it is just to make the time to listen to the complaint. This is difficult when you are busy, but making the complainant wait or passing them on to a more senior member of staff can escalate the situation (Robotham 2001).

- *Complainants want a reassurance that the organisation is taking the matter seriously and will try to prevent a recurrence*

    Do inform complainants what you intend to do about their complaint and how the trust will respond.

- *Complainants do not want to be told:*

    - that rules were being followed, so the organization was right all along.
    - that they made a mistake, so it is their own fault.

- detailed explanations of why a problem arose, which come across as an excuse for poor services.

⌘ ***It should be an objective to resolve as many complaints as possible at the first point of contact***

It is important that when a person complains, you try to handle it yourself in the first instance. Find out whether your employer provides training on complaints handling and ask to be sent for some. This can mean that you are better prepared to deal with complaints as they arise. However, if, after listening carefully, it becomes clear that you cannot resolve the issue or that it is a serious matter, you should inform the complainant about how to take the matter further.

If this is the first time you have had to deal with a complaint, make sure you seek support from your senior nurse or duty manager. You will not be expected to deal with a complaint by yourself, and the more senior staff will expect to be involved. Also, no matter how competently you deal with a complaint, some people will not be satisfied until they have spoken to someone 'in authority'. If your situation seems to be heading this way, don't see it as a failure – swallow your pride and call in a suitable member of staff.

Finally, do not forget to record the complaint and the action you took. Even if you feel that the complaint was dealt with immediately, the complainant may want to take things further at a later date. Clear records of the complaint, times and dates and the outcome will be vital if a formal investigation takes place.

How do I deal with aggressive patients or relatives?

There are occasions when a person will not complain in a reasonable manner but becomes verbally or physically aggressive. People may kick, punch, slap, bite or they may throw verbal insults or threats or make threatening gestures. All of these are considered to come under the broad heading of aggression (Garnham, 2001). As with many things, prevention is better than cure. It is important to be aware of the factors that may lead to aggression and act to reduce them.

Keeping people informed is particularly important as frustration can arise from anxiety and fear of the unknown, especially in strange environments such as hospitals. This may be made worse by the illness itself and the feelings of lack of control that patients or relatives may feel. For example, if there is time to be spent waiting to be seen by a member of staff it is important to keep going back every so often to apologize for the delay and explain why they may need to wait. In this situation, always be honest about the delay and do not try to invent an excuse, as this, if discovered, will only make the situation worse.

Spotting aggression before it happens and doing something to prevent it occurring is the ideal situation. However, this is not always possible, especially if the aggression is a result of alcohol, drugs or some altered state of consciousness and/or perception.

How should I deal with aggression when it happens?

Garnham (2001) recommends the use of the firefighting model. Basically this means identifying the elements that need to be present for a violent incident to occur and removing one of those elements.

Four elements are present in a violent incident:

- A target
- A weapon
- A trigger
- A state of arousal

Removing the target will usually mean that someone needs to leave the area. If it is another patient or relative you must gently persuade them that it is best to move away from the situation. Care needs to be taken here to ensure that you do not make yourself into the target. If you are the target for the aggression, withdrawing from the situation is likely to resolve the immediate problem, but may just mean that someone else becomes the target.

Removing a weapon that is being used can be impossible if it is a fist or a foot, and inadvisable if a knife or heavy object. You should on no account attempt to restrain or disarm someone unless you have received specific training to do this. You might ask the person to put the weapon down.

The trigger for the aggression may be easily removed if it is the behaviour of another person. But if the trigger is frustration over waiting times or the way that someone has just spoken to the aggressor, this cannot be removed once it has caused the aggression. Sometimes the trigger will seem to be trivial, but you need to remember that patients and relatives might already be in a heightened state of arousal as a result of the admission.

You may be able to reduce the state of arousal of the aggressive person. It is important to maintain eye contact (Garnham, 2001), but not to appear threatening by trying to stare the aggressor down. Speak calmly and be aware of body posture. You need to be assertive without being aggressive yourself. Without being patronising, do acknowledge the source of their frustration and anger. This can be done by simply saying something like 'I accept that this situation is frustrating for you but…' Let them know that their behaviour is making you uncomfortable or frightened (Garnham, 2001). You might try to appease the person by suggesting that you may be able to do something to resolve the situation. However, do not promise anything that cannot be delivered. For example, do not promise that you will get someone more senior to address the problem unless you can be fairly sure that the senior person will take some action.

You may not be able to do anything about the state of arousal of the aggressive person if they are under the influence of alcohol or drugs or in a confused state. If all else fails or you feel that you cannot personally deal with the situation, you should call for assistance. If you work in the community and are in a patient's house, you should leave the moment you feel in danger. If there are other people in the house that you feel might be attacked by the aggressive person, you should call the police.

Whatever the outcome of the situation, you should of course make clear and accurate records of what transpired, the action you took and the outcome of the incident (see below for incident reporting).

What is involved in incident reporting?

According to the Government's Chief Medical Officer, one in ten hospital patients suffer some accidental harm (*British Journal of Nursing*, 2002). Your immediate response to the incident is important. Clearly the priority is to ensure that anyone actually hurt receives prompt attention for their injuries. Green (2001) notes some confusion regarding how to respond when an incident occurs. Where an incident occurs that may lead to a claim against a nurse, the Royal College of Nursing advises:

> *'A member should never admit responsibility for any incident, or submit to the employer or to solicitors a written statement of the circumstances of the incident, until such report has been cleared by insurers through RCN Legal Services.'*
> (Royal College of Nursing, 2002)

It is likely that other professional indemnity schemes will contain similar advice. This advice is contrary to the stated aims for the management of clinical risk in the NHS (Green, 2001). One of these aims is for staff to be able to listen, apologize and learn from their mistakes.

So what do you do when faced with an incident? Do you apologize or seek union advice? Green (2001) advises that a nurse should not rush to apologize for an incident, but should record the facts, ensure that the line manager is made aware of the incident promptly and cooperate with the complaints procedure. Green (2001) suggests that when the investigation has been completed may be an appropriate point at which to apologize without compromising any indemnity insurance you may have.

It is clear that all incidents leading to harm, whether minor or major, must be reported (Department of Health, 2001f). Any incidents that nearly led to some harm (near misses) must also be reported. Each employer will have local systems for reporting incidents and near misses, and you should be familiar with the system in operation in your own area.

There are minimum requirements for the recording of incidents. These are listed in *Box 2.1*

> **Box 2.1**
> **Essential details to record in an incident report**
>
> - What happened? (event or near miss description, severity of actual or potential harm, people and equipment involved)
> - Where did it happen? (location/specialty)
> - When did it happen (date and time)?
> - How did it happen (immediate or proximate cause(s))?
> - Why did it happen (underlying or root causes(s))?
> - What action was taken or proposed (immediate and longer term)?
> - What impact did the event have (harm to the organization, the patient, others)?
> - What factors did, or could have, minimised the impact of the event?
>
> (Department of Health, 2001f)

What do I write?

When writing the record it is important to note clear and unambiguous facts – what you saw or what others say they saw, not what you or they think happened.
For example, if a patient falls, do not write:

> *'Mrs Smith seemed to have fallen out of bed.'*

Instead, write:

> *'Mrs Smith was found lying on the floor next to her bed'.*

You can record what someone says, for example:

> *'Mrs Smith stated that she fell out of bed.'*

Where you do record what someone says, it important to make it clear that it is someone else's words by enclosing the statement in quotation marks. You should also write down the events in chronological order as this can help to clarify precisely what happened. Any witnesses to the event should make a statement, and if the witness is another patient, a relative or a junior member of staff, they may need advice on how to write what happened to ensure that they also report facts rather than what they think happened.

If any person was injured or there is a suspicion of injury as a result of the incident, a doctor should examine that person. You should ensure that the doctor carrying out such an examination records:
- the fact that the examination was carried out
- whether any injury was apparent
- any advice given to the injured person.

What are my responsibilities in reporting malpractice?

There are two types of situations that may lead you to report malpractice. The first relates specifically to those who names appear on a professional register, such as nurses and doctors, and is usually termed professional misconduct. The second is malpractice by anyone within the care area or concerns about poor standards.

Professional misconduct

Nurses are advised to discuss any concerns they have about a registered colleague with their employer in the first instance (NMC, 2003). *Box 2.2* lists the most common types of professional misconduct reported to the NMC. The General Medical Council (2002) offers slightly different advice, suggesting that if a doctor's behaviour is putting a patient at risk, this should be reported to the Council immediately and less serious cases should be dealt with locally in the first instance. Both organizations require complaints to be made in writing. Therefore, you need to be sure of your facts and give a clear factual account of your concerns. That means stating what has actually occurred rather than what you suspect may have occurred. If you can get other witnesses to support your concerns, all the better. If there are no other witnesses, record all the facts including date and time and precisely what you observed. Remember to write down what you saw, not what you think happened.

Many nurses are afraid to report poor standards and malpractice, because of the potential for recriminations and possibly even loss of their job (O'Dowd, 2002). Certainly students that I teach often say they would be unlikely to complain about poor standards of care that they witness, out of fear of being failed in practice by their assessor as a reprisal. This culture of fear of reprisals seems to persist for the qualified nurse (Nazarko, 1998; *Health Which*, 1999; Wallis, 2001). This appears to remain the case in spite of the enactment of the

---

Box 2.2
Most common types of professional misconduct reported to the NMC

- Physical, sexual or verbal abuse of patients
- Stealing from patients
- Failing to care for patients properly (for employers and managers who are registered with the NMC, this can include failing to maintain an acceptable environment of care)
- Failing to keep proper records
- Failing to administer medicines safely
- Deliberately concealing unsafe practice
- Committing criminal offences

(Nursing & Midwifery Council, 2004b)

Public Interest Disclosure Act 1998, which protects the whistleblower if victimised or dismissed as a result of disclosing malpractice.

To whom should I report malpractice?

Under the Public Interest Disclosure Act 1998, protection from victimization and dismissal by an employer is given to those who speak out against any malpractice. Areas covered by the Public Interest Disclosure Act 1998 are listed in *Box 2.3*. However, this does not give carte blanche for anyone to go directly to the press with a complaint. All other reasonable attempts should be made to rectify a situation before going to the media. You should first raise any concerns internally with your employer, and if no progress is made you may take those concerns to a prescribed regulator; only then, if no progress is made, should concerns be raised externally to your employer. You are, however, allowed to seek legal advice and still be protected by the Act. If you decide to go to the media in the first instance, there is likely to be less protection from some sanctions, such as dismissal by your employer.

Box 2.3
Malpractice covered by the Public Interest Disclosure Act 1998

- Financial malpractice
- Criminal act, e.g. stealing, physical assault
- A danger to health and safety, e.g. where you or a colleague may not be fit to practise for reasons of health or competence
- Where the environment jeopardises standards of practice, e.g. a lack of resources, where staffing levels are unsafe
- Any damage to the environment
- A failure to comply with a legal obligation, e.g. negligence, breach of contract, breach of administrative law
- A miscarriage of justice
- An attempt to cover up any of the above

(Royal College of Nursing, 2002)

Reporting malpractice internally

Concerns should first be raised with your employer, such as your line manager, senior colleague or supervisor. For example, if you are a staff nurse then you should raise the issue with the charge nurse or more senior nurse. If the person you have concerns about is your manager and you work in the NHS, you have the right to raise concerns with the trust board, the health authority or even a health minister (Royal College of Nursing, 2002).

Prescribed regulator

If you work in the independent sector, such as a nursing home or private hospital, concerns can be raised with a prescribed regulator. Regulators include the Health and Safety Executive, the Inland Revenue, the Audit Commission and the local authority. You may also report concerns to a prescribed regulator if you feel that those concerns have not been acted upon by an NHS employer.

Legal adviser

Should you need independent and confidential advice about a concern of malpractice, disclosures to a legal adviser are protected under the Act. This means that you can seek a legal opinion without being accused of breaching confidentiality.

Reporting malpractice externally

The Act does allow for reporting of malpractice to the police, media, MPs etc. under exceptional circumstances, i.e. where one of the following conditions is satisfied:

- Raised internally or with a prescribed person, but was not dealt with properly.
- Not raised internally or with a prescribed regulator, because the worker reasonably fears that he/she would be victimised.
- Not raised internally because the worker reasonably believes that there would be a cover-up and there is no prescribed person.

(Royal College of Nursing, 2002)

It may also be advisable to seek advice from a representative of your union. However, the law does give the greatest protection for internal disclosure, which includes reports made to government ministers. If you decided to take your concerns to the media before raising them with your employer, the Act would provide less protection from dismissal than if you had used the institution's grievance procedures. There is a good deal of useful advice on reporting malpractice on the Public Concern at Work website (http://www.pcaw.co.uk). *Box 2.4* lists some useful do's and don'ts suggested on this website.

What can I do about bullying within the organisation?

Bullying is increasingly being recognised as a problem. Indeed, a Royal College of Nursing survey revealed that up to one in six nurses are subject to bullying at work (Pearce, 2001). If you are being bullied, you will generally want it to stop. However, as a nurse you probably also have a professional duty to take action if you are aware that someone is being bullied. Although the NMC *Code*

Box 2.4 Whistleblowing do's and don'ts	
Do	❖ Keep calm ❖ Think about the risks and outcomes before you act ❖ Remember that you are a witness, not a complainant ❖ Phone us for advice on 020 7404 6609
Don't	❖ Forget there may be an innocent or good explanation ❖ Become a private detective ❖ Use a whistleblowing procedure to pursue a personal grievance ❖ Expect thanks
	(Public Concern at Work, 2002)

of Professional Conduct (Nursing and Midwifery Council, 2004a) does not make explicit mention of bullying, it does state in clause 8.3 that there is a duty to report circumstances in the care environment that could jeopardise standards of practice. It would be hard to imagine anyone delivering a high standard of care if they are subject to bullying. There is probably also a duty placed on you by your employer through local policies which outline action that should be taken if you are aware of bullying.

How do you recognise when you or another member of staff is being bullied?

It is not always obvious when you are being bullied. Howells-Johnson (2000) defines bullying as persistent unwelcome behaviour, such as:

- unwarranted or invalid criticism
- nit-picking
- fault finding
- exclusion
- isolation of another
- singling someone out
- treating someone differently
- shouting at someone
- humiliating someone
- excessive monitoring of someone's work performance.

Other examples might include making unreasonable work demands on a person and inciting others to hold a negative opinion of someone.

What should you do?

The first thing to do is to recognise bullying behaviour for what it is. There can be no excuse for it, especially in the workplace. Any criticism of your or anyone else's performance should be constructive and based on facts, not destructive and based on conjecture or mere opinion. As with much of what is discussed in this chapter, record what is happening. According to Grove (2000) it is not the incident itself that necessarily counts, but the frequency and the regularity with which it happens. White (2002a) also suggests talking to colleagues about the bullying, as you might not be the only one. Alternatively, if it is not you that is being bullied, but a colleague, talking to others may reveal several team members who do not like the situation and are prepared to support you in taking action against the bully.

Your trust or employer should have anti-bullying policies in place. Find out what they are and use them to take action. Dimond (2002) points out that your employer has a legal duty under health and safety law to protect employees from bullying. Additionally, under article 3 of the Human Rights Act 1998, you have the right to freedom from inhuman and degrading treatment. It is inhuman and degrading to bully someone and the employer has a clear duty to prevent this abuse of human rights. You also have legal protection under the Public Interest Disclosure Act 1998 if you blow the whistle and report an employer for bullying (see section on reporting malpractice above).

You should be aware of the potentially detrimental effects that bullying can have on your health and should seek medical advice if you feel that your health is affected. If you are off sick as a result of bullying, record it in the accident book at work. If necessary, you can take out a grievance against the bully through your employer's grievance procedures. Human resources or personnel departments should be able to give advice and support in this.

Your union representative should also be able to offer advice and guidance on handling the situation. Several case studies of bullying reported in the press indicate that the victims felt embarrassed about being a victim and suffered in silence until they were driven out of their job. The key is not to suffer alone but to share your feelings with others and report bullying behaviour. Grove (2000) goes as far as suggesting that if the bully is aggressive in public, you should get a solicitor's letter sent to the bully with regard to the slander or defamation of character. The most important thing is not to allow the bully to win by forcing a change in your behaviour or moving jobs. Not only will your self-esteem take a serious blow, but the bully is likely to move on to another target. You should not have to pay the price for someone else's unacceptable behaviour.

What do I do if a patient wants to self-discharge?

All patients, unless detained under the Mental Health Act, are voluntary and cannot be kept in hospital or a nursing/residential home against their will. You have a professional duty to ensure the safety and wellbeing of people who lack the capacity to make decisions for themselves. Thus, if a person lacks that capacity and is intending to self-discharge, it may be necessary to consider seeking a psychiatric referral.

If, on the other hand, there is no evidence of any lack of capacity, any person over the age of 18 years has the right to decide for themselves whether to accept or reject medical advice, including whether to remain in hospital. Merely wanting to discharge oneself against medical advice is not evidence of lack of capacity to make a rational decision.

It is preferable that persons wishing to discharge themselves sign a written declaration that they are taking self-discharge against medical advice. Your employer should have forms for this specific purpose. However, there is no legal requirement that the patient actually signs the form. So what can you do if a patient decides to self-discharge and refuses to sign the declaration/form? Recording the event is imperative. Some indication of the patient's reasons for self-discharge might be helpful. However, the essential facts that must be recorded are the time and date the patient left. It is also important to record any advice that was given to the patient by yourself or anyone else.

What advice should you give? If the patient is willing to listen, you should consider informing them:

- why it is best to remain in hospital
- the potential health consequences of taking self-discharge at that point in their care
- that they should inform their own GP
- that the consultant will probably inform their GP
- how to continue their care at home
- when to seek help from a medical practitioner
- the telephone number of NHS Direct
- the hospital/ward contact number.

It might also be useful to consider producing a leaflet outlining general advice regarding self-discharge if your institution does not already have one. You should, of course, ensure that if the medical staff do not already know, they are informed immediately of the situation.

How do I deal with MRSA?

Antibiotic-resistant bacteria are a constant worry in the health service. The papers regularly report outbreaks of 'superbugs'. So how should you tackle this problem? Methicillin-resistant *Staphylococcus aureus* (MRSA) has existed since 1968 in America and it is estimated that 50% of all hospital-acquired *S. aureus* infections are methicillin resistant (Sheff, 2003). The most common source of staphylococcal infections appears to be the nasal passages of individuals, although there are reports of high levels of bacteria and fungal spores, including MRSA, in hospital mattresses, chairs and other furniture (White, 2002b).

As yet, there is no effective way of eliminating these bacteria (van Belkum and Verbrugh, 2001). Therefore, preventing their spread and dealing effectively with outbreaks are particularly important.

How do I prevent the spread of MRSA?

In addition to the specific recommendations shown in *Box 2.5* for hospital patients, and *Box 2.6* for residents of nursing and residential homes, there are a number of things you can do to help prevent the spread of MRSA.

- Carry out regular audits of handwashing to ensure that staff are adhering to policies.
- Encourage the use of moisturisers to eliminate cracked or chapped skin as this can discourage handwashing.
- Use waterless hand sanitisers where there is no visible soiling of hands as this can also help to prevent drying and cracking of skin.
- Ensure effective cleaning of any shared equipment.
- Liaise with the infection control team.

Box 2.5
Recommendations for preventing the spread of MRSA in hospital patients

- Scrupulous handwashing by hospital staff before and after contact with patients and before any procedure.
- Patients with MRSA should be physically isolated in a single room with the door remaining closed and the room regularly damp dusted, or they should be nursed in a special ward away from other non-infected patients.
- The patient's notes should be clearly labelled.
- The use of antibiotics, such as those applied inside the nose (mupirocin), and bathing (with antiseptic soap) will also help to reduce the risk of spread.
- Finally, when such a patient is discharged from hospital, his/her room should be comprehensively cleaned and all linen and other clinical waste disposed of in special bags.

(Association of Medical Microbiologists, 2002)

The Department of Health (1996) provides specific guidance for nursing and residential homes in dealing with MRSA (*Box 2.6*).

If a patient in your care is diagnosed as having MRSA, the precautions listed above should be applied. If several patients are diagnosed an investigation should be commenced to identify any potential cause of the cross-infection, such as shared equipment or staff who may be carriers. The infection control team will be an invaluable source of help and guidance in such instances.

Final points

Remember that if a patient cannot mobilise and is confined to a side room with a label of 'infectious', he/she is probably going to feel isolated and possibly stigmatised. You can help the patient by encouraging visitors to stagger the

> **Box 2.6**
> **Guidance on caring for nursing/residential home residents with MRSA**
>
> ❖ Those with MRSA should be helped with handwashing if their mental or physical condition makes it difficult for them to wash their hands for themselves. They should be encouraged to live a normal life without restriction and they need not be isolated.
>
> ❖ They may share a room so long as neither they nor the person with whom they are sharing has open sores or wounds, infusions or catheters.
>
> ❖ They may join other residents in communal areas, such as sitting or dining rooms, so long as any sores or wounds are covered with an appropriate dressing, which is changed regularly.
>
> ❖ They may receive visitors and go out of the home, e.g. to see their family or friends.
>
> (Department of Health, 1996)

times of their visits. Make sure that the patient understands his/her condition and is not isolated unless absolutely essential. All trusts will have an infection control nurse or team, who will be an invaluable source of information and support to the ward staff and the patient.

How do I deal with the unexpected?
Personal notes and contacts

Chapter 3

What principles do practical nursing skills involve?

- What is the essential role of the nurse?
- What are the principles of caring for patients with wound drains?
- How do I look after a nasogastric or gastric tube?
- What is the nursing management of intravenous therapy?
- What is involved in catheterisation and catheter care?
- What is a syringe driver?
- How do I monitor central venous pressure?
- What do I need to know about different wound dressings?
- What does an aseptic technique involve?
- What are the principles of preparing patients for tests and investigations?
- How can I promote continence?
- What are the most common signs of a urinary tract infection?
- What do I need to know about pressure ulcers?
- How do I help my patients meet their nutritional needs?

What is the essential role of the nurse?

Penny Tremayne

The so-called 'basics' of nursing care, such as food and nutrition, continence/bladder care and pressure ulcers, are essential and fundamental, as highlighted by the Department of Health (2001a). Patients with acute, chronic and ongoing healthcare needs may, at some point, become compromised for one reason or another, and will often require nursing interventions in these three aspects of care. Your role as a nurse will include:

- Assessment: identifying actual or potential patient problems on an ongoing basis.
- Planning: setting achievable goals and subsequent prescription of an individualised care plan.
- Implementation: delivering or facilitating delivery of a prescribed, individualised care plan.
- Evaluation: judging and monitoring the effectiveness of the care delivered.
- Maintaining the dignity, respect and trust of individual patients.
- Benchmarking: comparing and sharing best practice (Department of Health, 2001a).
- Self-care: maximising patient independence.
- Record keeping – maintaining ongoing, accurate records.

What are the principles of caring for patients with wound drains?
Nicola Brooks

Wound drains are widely used within the clinical setting to aid the removal of fluid, such as exudate, blood, pus and other body fluids that may collect in cavities or dead spaces within a wound (Torrance and Maylor, 1999). The accumulation of fluid within the wound bed increases the risk of infection, so it is important to remove the static fluid in order to aid healing (Smith *et al*, 1999).

There are a variety of wound drains available, but they all work by one of two mechanisms: passive drainage, using gravity to release the fluid into a collecting bag or dressing (e.g. corrugated drains, tube drains); or active drainage, using a vacuum or suction mechanism to remove the fluid.

Wound drains are used for three main reasons:

- therapeutic drainage
- prophylactic drainage
- decompressive drainage.

- *Therapeutic drainage* is used to remove infected material such as bacteria, pus or dead tissue from the body, or to reduce the dead space within a wound to prevent abscess formation. Surgical techniques used for therapeutic drainage include needle aspiration, incision and drainage, and complete surgical excision.

- *Prophylactic drainage* is used to prevent infection, but this practice has been replaced by the use of antibiotic therapy and has now largely been abandoned.

- *Decompressive drainage* is intended to prevent leakage of urine, bile, intestinal and pancreatic fluid, or to prevent fluid accumulating either within or around the wound, to reduce the risk of further complications.

Complications of wound drains

There are relatively few complications associated with wound drains. However, Dougherty and Simmons (1992) have identified a few risks:

- the drain is a 'foreign body', which may impair healing
- perforation
- inflammation
- movement or misplacement of the drain
- kinking or obstruction of the tubing
- breakage or accidental removal
- pain
- tissue ingrowth
- fluid and electrolyte loss.

Nursing management of drains

Observation and careful handling of wound drains are paramount within the practice setting. There are many factors that should be taken into account when caring for a patient with a drain in situ.

- **Monitoring the drain/drainage fluid**
  The colour, amount, and nature of the drainage fluid should be recorded onto the fluid balance/wound drainage chart. Excessive drainage or changes in the type of fluid (particularly fresh blood) should be recorded and reported to the medical team.

- **Observation of the drain/drain site**
  Observe the drain site for damage to the surrounding skin caused by inflammation or fluid exudate. Gloves should be used when handling drains or the drainage system. Check that the drain system is well secured with no kinks or obstruction of the tubing that may hinder the drainage process. Check that the suture(s) are secure and not pulling the skin.

- **Patient information**
  Ensure that the patient is kept fully informed of why the drain is there and how long it will need to remain in place, in order to reduce anxiety, as well as provide practical assistance on teaching the patient how to cope with a drain. To ensure compliance, factors such as ensuring that the drain remains patent, effective and aseptic, and how the drain will be removed, should be explained to the patient. Patients who are mobile may be uncomfortable with the image that the drain portrays. This is particularly important in women having surgery for breast cancer. In these circumstances it may be possible to 'disguise' the drain bag as a small handbag.

Removing a drain

1. Explain the procedure fully to the patient and ask him/her to get into a comfortable position before removal of the drain.
2. Check the medical notes to ensure that the drain is to be removed.
3. If the drain is on an active drainage system (the vacuumed/suction method), de-vacuum the drain to reduce trauma to the tissues as the drain is pulled out.
4. Wash hands and apply sterile gloves. Maintain an aseptic technique during the procedure (see section on aseptic technique).
5. Cut the retaining suture.
6. Gently and smoothly remove the drain (difficulty in removing the drain may indicate adhesions, so always seek medical advice if you are unsure).
7. Apply a sterile dressing to the drain site, and observe for bleeding/leakage.
8. Dispose of all equipment appropriately (drains are clinical waste).
9. Document the procedure in the nursing notes.

Changing a vacuum drainage system bottle

It may be necessary to change the drainage bottle if the drain is yielding large amounts, or if there is a loss of vacuum to the drainage system.

1. Explain the procedure fully to the patient.
2. Wash hands, put on sterile gloves.
3. Clamp drainage tubing near to drainage site and bottle.
4. Disconnect bottle and wipe with an alcohol-impregnated swab to ensure that it is an aseptic procedure.
5. Connect new bottle to the tubing.
6. Unclamp both clamps.
7. Ensure that the drain is patent and drainage fluid is coming down the tube.
8. Remember to document drainage fluid measurements on the fluid balance chart or wound drainage chart.

How do I look after a nasogastric or gastric tube?
Nicola Brooks and Penny Tremayne

Nasogastric tubes are used for four main reasons:

- **Before or following abdominal surgery:** To ensure that the stomach is empty, and to relieve any anastomosis (artificial connection of internal structures) of pressure.

- **Persistent vomiting:** To reduce the risk of aspiration and ensure patient comfort.

- **Intestinal obstruction:** To empty the stomach and to ensure patient comfort.

- **Short- or long-term feeding:** For individuals who are not able to meet their nutritional requirements but have a functioning gastrointestinal tract.

Inserting a nasogastric tube

Equipment required

- Nasogastric tube of appropriate size and type, e.g. Ryles tube, fine-bore tube (fine-bore tubes are *only* used for feeding purposes)
- Lubricant (water-soluble jelly or water)
- Litmus paper/pH paper to check the position of the nasogastric tube
- Receiver/vomit bowl
- 10 ml syringe
- Clinical waste bag, tissues, tape to secure tube in position
- Spigot or drainage bag as necessary
- Non-sterile gloves.

Procedure

1. Explain the procedure to the patient and gain consent.
2. Take all the equipment to the bedside and ensure patient privacy.
3. Wash hands and put on gloves.
4. Ensure that the patient is sitting comfortably – ideally sitting upright.
5. Estimate the length of tube to be passed by measuring the distance from the nose to the earlobe, and down to the xiphisternum. Use your second hand to hold the correct position, or use the markers on the nasogastric tube as guidance.
6. Select the best nostril to insert the tube into (not tender, no deviated septum etc). Ask the patient to blow his/her nose or sniff through each nostril to establish the most patent nostril.
7. Encourage the patient to relax and to breathe normally.
8. Lubricate the tip of the nasogastric tube.
9. Pass the tube gently into the nostril, and pass backwards to the nasopharynx (if you experience difficulty in passing the tube, remove it and try the other nostril).
10. Check patient comfort and allow patient to recover for a few minutes.
11. Ask the patient to breathe through the mouth and swallow. At the point of swallowing, gently advance the tube into the stomach to the required length. (A sip of water given when passing the tube may assist swallowing).
12. Check the position of the tube in the stomach by one of the following methods:

    - Aspirate stomach contents with a 10 ml syringe. Check to see whether the litmus paper has turned pink to indicate gastric acidity. If using pH paper, check that the pH is less than 4.0 (University Hospitals of Leicester Nutrition Support Team, 2002).
    - Insert 5–10 ml of air into the tube while another nurse listens to the stomach with a stethoscope. As air enters the stomach, a gurgling sound will be heard (this technique is not used in children).
    - X-ray to check the position (this is not necessary with a Ryles tube; however, fine-bore feeding tubes have a guidewire in place, which will show on X-ray).

13. Secure the tube in position with tape.

Potential problems following insertion of a nasogastric tube

- **No aspirate**: If no aspirate occurs, ensure that the tube is in the correct position by checking the back of the throat for coiling. If the tube is coiled, try to re-position it slightly and re-aspirate.

- **Tube misplacement:** This is often indicated by respiratory distress or coughing. If the patient is showing signs of respiratory distress, this probably indicates that the nasogastric tube has entered the respiratory passage, and the tube should be removed immediately.

- **Unable to pass tube past nasal cavity:** Ask the patient for suggestions as to why the tube may not pass, e.g. previous nasal surgery, injury. Try the other nostril. If you are still unable to pass the tube, then leave alone.

How do I know if the nasogastric tube is in the correct position?

Make sure you check your local policy/protocol for any specific details. Gastric aspirate on pH-sensitive paper strips should confirm the position of the tube.

- pH 3–4 indicates gastric position.
- pH >6 indicates bronchial positioning. The patient may also become distressed by coughing or gagging and appear cyanosed.
- pH 6–8 indicates that the tube has passed through the stomach into the intestine (aspirate will be green/yellow, indicating the presence of bile. Note also whether the patient is receiving medication (e.g. antacids, proton pump inhibitors) that can cause changes in the gastric pH (Burnham, 2000). If in any doubt at all, then do not commence feeding until position has been confirmed by X-ray.

What should I be specifically looking for when nursing a patient with a gastrostomy?

- Check your local policy/protocol for specific details.
- Check the site of the gastrostomy for redness, inflammation or pain. A dressing should only be in place for the initial 24 hours (Howell, 2002).
- Check that the tube can be rotated 360° to prevent scar tissue formation (Howell, 2002).
- If there is pain, bleeding, signs of perforation, aspiration or that the gastrostomy has been pulled out, seek medical and specialist nurse assistance immediately.

What can I do to prevent the nasogastric/gastrostomy tube becoming blocked?

- Flush the tube with water regularly, before and after every feed and before and after each drug administration (Colagiovanni, 2000; Bryson, 2001).
- Use a polyurethane nasogastric tube (Colagiovanni, 2000).

Can I administer drugs via a nasogastric/gastrostromy tube?

- Apply local policy/protocol.
- Yes you can, but you should always seek the advice of the pharmacist as there are factors that can affect drug interaction, drug dosage and method of delivery, which you need to consider (Bryson, 2001).

What should I do if the tube is blocked?

- Make sure that you check the local policy/protocol for specific details.
- Flush tube with warm sterile water.
- Milk the tube with fingers to aid 'unclogging' of the tube. There is some debate regarding the use of carbonated drinks and pancreatic enzymes, but the evidence supporting this is inconclusive, and in this instance you should be advised by medical or specialist nurse staff.

What is the nursing management of intravenous therapy?
Nicola Brooks

If a patient is unable to tolerate enough oral fluids to maintain a sufficient fluid balance, intravenous (IV) therapy will be required. This may be given on either a short-term basis, e.g. postoperatively until oral intake is resumed, or for several days if the patient is being kept nil by mouth.

The most common reasons for using IV therapy are:

- dehydration
- vomiting and/or diarrhoea
- excessive insensible loss (e.g. sweating)
- preoperative and postoperative hydration
- hypercatabolism
- unconsciousness.

Nursing management of an IV infusion

The basic principles of caring for an IV infusion are:

- Wash hands and maintain aseptic conditions when dealing with the infusion.
- Maintain a closed system.
- Ensure that the packaging for the fluid to be infused is not damaged, and the fluid's 'use by date' is still current.
- Ensure that fluids hang no longer than 24 hours (4 hours for blood) as some solutions deteriorate in bright sunlight.
- Ensure that the cannula site is clean and dry, and checked on a regular basis for signs of infection, and that the cannula is held securely to the patient. It is recommended that a cannula should be re-sited after 72 hours (Centers for Disease Control, 1982), but this may vary according to local policy.
- Infusion sets should be changed every 48–72 hours (Maki and Ringer, 1987). It is good practice to record the date and time that the set is due to be changed.
- Ensure that infusion rates are maintained accurately.
- Record and monitor an accurate fluid balance.

In order to avoid complications with the administration of IV infusions, it is important that the correct site, cannula size and infusion device are used. An IV cannula is normally inserted into a peripheral vein by a member of the medical team, but can be inserted by nursing staff as part of an expanded/extended role. The appropriate size of cannula to be inserted depends on such factors as the volume and type of fluid to be infused, the duration of IV therapy, the ease of access and the patency of peripheral veins. It is also important to check which arm the patient would like the cannula sited in, wherever possible, as this may increase compliance. The non-dominant arm is recommended. For cannulae that are to be inserted within the wrist or antecubital fossa, a splint may be required for support and to prevent flexion.

A wealth of infusion sets is available, but the set commonly used in the clinical setting contains a valve mechanism designed to prevent air entry if the infusion fluid runs out. These also have a macro-drip system, which takes approximately 15–20 drops for every one millilitre (ml) of fluid. The number of drops per millilitre is variable depending on the viscosity of the fluid: approximately 15 drops for blood and high viscosity fluids, and approximately 20 drops for clear fluids.

Where smaller volumes of fluid are to be infused, or a more precise rate of flow control is required, the use of a volumetric infusion control pump device is recommended. Blood and blood products are given via blood administration sets, which are discarded either immediately after completion of the transfusion, after 12 hours of first use, or if the filter becomes blocked, but this may vary according to local policy.

Calculating flow control

It is important to ensure that the type of fluid, the volume, infusion time, date and signature of the prescriber are documented on the fluid prescription sheet. It is the nurse's responsibility to calculate the flow rate and ensure that the correct rate is maintained. A formula is used to calculate the correct flow rate (Galford, 1990); however, it is essential to know the number of drops per millilitre (ml) being delivered by the infusion set. (Standard infusion sets normally give approximately 15–20 drops/ml of fluid infused.)

$$\frac{\text{No. of millilitres to be infused}}{\text{No. of hours over which the infusion is to be delivered}} \times \frac{\text{No. of drops per ml}}{\text{60 minutes}} = \text{No. of drops delivered per minute}$$

Example

A 1000 ml bag of fluid to be delivered over 8 hours, using a standard infusion set (delivering 20 drops/ml), would work out as:

$$\frac{1000}{8} \times \frac{20}{60} = \textbf{42 drops per minute}$$

Remember…

Certain factors (see list below) affect the flow rate, so the infusion needs to be checked regularly to ensure that it is running continuously. There should be no alterations to 'catch up' the infusion regimen.

- Cannula position, movement or patency
- Problems with the infusion equipment, e.g. blocked filters, kinked tubing, height of fluid container
- Infusion fluid factors, e.g. viscosity, temperature, specific gravity
- Complications of venous spasm, e.g. infiltration, phlebitis, thrombophlebitis.

Complications of infusion therapy (Speechley and Toovey, 1987)

- **Infiltration and extravasation**
  This occurs when the infusion fluid leaks into the tissues as a result of the cannula or needle becoming displaced. There may be oedema at the site, the patient may complain of pain and the skin around the site may feel cooler than the surrounding skin. If the fluid or additive is a vesicant, then this can cause tissue necrosis.

- **Infection at the insertion site – phlebitis and thrombophlebitis:**
  Inflammation of the vein is termed phlebitis; thrombophlebitis occurs when inflammation is further complicated by the formation of a blood clot within the vein. Phlebitis and thrombophlebitis may be caused by movement of the cannula within the vein, or by contaminated equipment or fluids. Both phlebitis and thrombophlebitis can be minimised by attention to technique and good infection control measures.

What is involved in catheterisation and catheter care?
Nicola Brooks and Penny Tremayne

Catheterisation is the insertion of a special tube into the bladder, using an aseptic technique, for the purpose of evacuating or instilling fluids (Dougherty and Lister, 2002). Stickler and Zimakoff (1994) and Winn (1998) consider that the use of a catheter should be avoided if at all possible, so ask yourself: have all possible strategies been exhausted?

When is catheterisation likely to be considered?

- Postoperatively: to accurately monitor urine output.
- In acute illness: e.g. post-myocardial infarction or heart failure.
- For urinary retention: e.g. postoperatively or enlarged prostate gland.
- For urinary incontinence: as a last resort and only after full investigation and implementation of other management strategies.

- In the terminally ill or unconscious: to prevent possible breakdown in skin integrity.
- Others: for determination of residual urine volume; to empty the bladder before investigation; teaching intermittent self-catheterisation; and intravesical instillation of drugs (Stewart, 2001).

Catheterisation may be carried out for the following reasons:

- To empty the bladder preoperatively or postoperatively and before specific investigations
- To relieve urine retention
- To determine residual urine
- To measure accurate urine output
- To bypass obstruction
- To relieve incontinence (when there is no other practicable means).

A guide to catheters and catheter materials

There is a wide range of catheters available; careful assessment of the correct size and appropriate material will help to minimise complications. The main criterion for the selection of an appropriate catheter material is considered to be the length of time the catheter is expected to remain in place (see below for types of catheters in use). The time scales for catheter use are:

- Short term: 1–21 days
- Short to medium term: 2–6 weeks
- Medium to long term: 6 weeks to 3 months

The size of catheter to be inserted should be the smallest necessary to maintain adequate drainage (McGill, 1982). Laurent (1998) suggests that, provided that the urine is clear, the general rule for catheter size is as follows:

- Adult female: 12–14 Charriere (Ch) gauge
- Adult male: 12–16 Ch gauge.

The use of a larger gauge catheter can have side-effects, such as discomfort for the patient, or pressure sores and abscess formation. Larger gauge catheters may be appropriate if there are blood clots or debris in the urine (Stewart, 2001).

- The length of the catheter should be appropriate. Female catheters are shorter than male catheters and therefore pull less, hence they are more comfortable. However, if a female patient is confined to bed, then the extra length of a male catheter gives better drainage.
- A size 12–14 Ch gauge is usually sufficient.
- Consider a larger catheter (16–18 Ch) if there is mucus or debris in the urine.
- Consider a size 18 Ch or greater if haematuria and clots are present.

What type of catheter should be inserted?

- **Latex:** Latex is purified rubber, which is soft and flexible. However, plain latex can quickly become encrusted and cause urethral trauma (Laurent, 1998). Latex should only be used for short-term catheterisation. Make sure you check the allergy status of the patient first.
- **Teflon/silicone coated:** This is a coating applied to a standard latex catheter, to reduce urethral irritation. These catheters are recommended for short- to medium-term catheterisation.
- **Silicone**: Catheters made from silicone are used for long-term catheterisation. They have a wider lumen, and are less likely to become blocked.
- **Hydrogel coated:** Hydrogel catheters are made from latex covered with a hydrophilic polymer coating, which is considered to cause minimum irritation to the urethra. These catheters are recommended for long-term use.

Table 3.1 summarises the length of time that catheters may remain in place.

Table 3.1. How long can a catheter stay in place?		
Type	Duration	Catheter material
Short term	Up to 3 weeks	• Plastic • Latex • Teflon-coated polytetrafluoroethylene (PTFE Teflon) • Silicone elastomer
Medium term	Up to 6 weeks	• PTFE Teflon • Silicone elastomer
Long term	Up to 12 weeks	• Pure silicone • Hydrogel

Inserting a urinary catheter

Equipment required

- Catheterisation pack (contains towels, galipot, receiver, swabs)
- Disposable pad
- Sterile gloves (two pairs) and apron
- Appropriate catheter
- Local anaesthetic and lubricating gel (for both genders)
- Normal saline (for cleaning the site)
- Syringe and sterile normal saline or water (to inflate catheter balloon)
- Catheter drainage bag.

Procedure

1. Explain the procedure to the patient and gain consent.
2. Take all of the equipment to the bedside and ensure patient privacy.

3. Female patients are best placed in a supine position with knees bent, hips flexed and feet resting apart (they may keep covered at this stage). Male patients can lie in a comfortable position as their condition dictates.
4. Wash hands, put on disposable apron.
5. Prepare the trolley: open equipment packs, placing the equipment required on the top shelf.
6. Position a disposable pad under the patient's buttocks to ensure that urine does not leak onto the bedclothes.
7. Wash hands. Put on two pairs of gloves.
8. Place sterile towels across the patient's thighs, and the receiver tray between the patient's legs to collect urine.
9. *Female catheterisation*: Separate the labia minora and clean around the urethral orifice with swabs, using single downward strokes. Insert the nozzle of the lubricating jelly into the urethra and squeeze out the content. Remove one pair of gloves.
   Male catheterisation: Wrap a swab around the penis (retracting the foreskin if necessary) and clean the glans penis with normal saline. Insert the nozzle of the lubricating jelly into the urethra and squeeze out the content. Massage the gel along the urethra. Remove one pair of gloves.
10. *Female catheterisation*: Insert the tip of the catheter into the urethral orifice in an upward and backward direction. Advance for approximately 5 cm until urine is detected.
    Male catheterisation: Grasp the shaft of the penis, raising it until it is extended. Insert the catheter slowly for approximately 20 cm, until urine flows.
11. Inflate the balloon according to the manufacturer's instructions (normally approx 10 ml normal saline).
12. Withdraw the catheter slightly and connect to the drainage system.
13. Ensure patient comfort, and that the area is clean and dry.
14. Measure the amount of urine yielded.
15. Dispose of all equipment in a clinical waste bag.
16. Document all details relating to the procedure (catheter type and batch number, size, balloon size, date) in the nursing notes.

What do I do if the catheter is not draining any urine and appears to be blocked or is leaking?

Check initially for the following:

1. Catheter and drainage tubing are not kinked
2. The catheter drainage bag is below bladder level
3. The catheter drainage bag is not full
4. There is no other obstruction, such as occlusion of the inlet valve by the strap of a leg bag
5. The patient is not constipated, as pressure on the drainage lumen can prevent the catheter from draining (Pomfret, 1999; Rew and Woodward, 2001).

A common method for unblocking a catheter is a 'bladder washout'; however, as Evans and Godfrey (2001) highlight, its efficacy is debatable and the use of such terminology is confusing. At present, it appears that the nurse should do what he/she can to prevent the blockage of a catheter. This includes:

- Ensuring that the patient maintains a high or at least recommended fluid intake (Wells, 1998;s Pomfret, 1999; Godfrey and Evans, 2001).
- Encouraging the patient to drink cranberry juice (Nazarko, 1995; Leaver, 1996; Lavender, 2000).
- Monitoring urine pH for alkalinity at least weekly or more frequently (Gates, 2000; Rew, 2001). Burr and Nuseibeh (1997) found that catheters block more often when the urine has a high pH, so aim to keep the pH below 6.8.
- Monitoring the life of the catheter for each individual patient.
- Changing the catheter before blockage can occur.
- Optimum management of a frequently blocked catheter is to change it – check old catheter tip for encrustations on removal (Wells, 1998).
- Informing medical staff: detrusor instability is a possibility and an anticholinergic may need to be prescribed.
- A bladder washout can be considered in patients with long-term catheters; refer to local guidelines and/or policies.

Removing a catheter

If possible, catheters should normally be removed at night or in the early morning, so that any urine retention problems can be dealt with during the day.

Equipment required

- Disposable gloves (non-sterile)
- Syringe for deflating balloon (normally 10 ml)
- Clinical waste bag
- Urine measuring jug.

Procedure

1. Explain the procedure to the patient and gain consent. Inform the patient of any potential problems that may occur after removal of the catheter (e.g. urgency, frequency or discomfort from irritation of the urethra by the catheter).
2. Empty the residual content of urine in the drainage bag into a measuring jug and chart accordingly on the fluid balance chart.
3. Wash your hands and put on gloves.
4. Use syringe to deflate the balloon (see below if a problem occurs)
5. Ask the patient to relax, and slowly breathe in and out. On exhalation, gently, but quickly, remove the catheter.
6. Clean the patient, and make him/her comfortable.
7. Dispose of all equipment in a clinical waste bag.

What should I do if a catheter balloon will not deflate?

- Look for the obvious again. Is there anything obstructing the catheter tubing? Is it kinked? Is there faecal impaction?
- Is there encrustation that may be dissolved by a catheter maintenance solution?
- Is the syringe that you are using faulty? Try another one.
- Leave the syringe in situ to drain spontaneously.
- Next, attach a needle to a 10 ml syringe and insert the needle into the side arm of the catheter (above the inflation valve) and drain water gently.
- Inform medical staff if the catheter balloon still cannot be deflated (Rew and Woodward, 2001).

What is a syringe driver?

Nicola Brooks

A syringe driver is a portable battery-operated infusion pump that delives drugs via a continuous subcutaneous route at a predetermined rate (Dougherty and Lister, 2002). It should be used for patients who are unable to tolerate medication via an oral route, and has become a well-established technique for delivering analgesia, antiemetics and sedatives (Coyle, 1986)

The advantages of using a syringe driver are listed in *Box 3.1*. There are very few disadvantages to using this type of device. However, the nurse must be sure which type of device is being used – a 12-hour or 24-hour one – in order to determine the correct flow rate. Before setting up an infusion device, you must be familiar with the correct operational technique. Also, the cannula and skin site need to be selected carefully, as infection and inflammation may occur.

Box 3.1
Advantages of using a syringe driver

- Avoids the administration of intermittent injections
- Allows a mixture of drugs to be given together (subject to drug compatibility)
- Ensures accurate infusion times
- Syringe drivers are lightweight and portable, which makes them ideal for use in the community setting or for ambulatory infusions
- Drugs are delivered over a 12- or 24-hour period (depending on the device used)

Selection of infusion sites

Recommended sites for continuous infusion are the lateral aspects of the upper arms and thighs, abdomen, anterior chest below the clavicle and the back (although this is only very occasionally used) (Nicholson, 1986). A winged infusion set is used, commonly known as a 'butterfly' line. The procedure for inserting a butterfly line is outlined in *Box 3.2*.

> **Box 3.2**
> **Insertion of a butterfly line**
>
> 1. Explain the procedure and gain the patient's consent.
> 2. Assist the patient in adopting a comfortable position.
> 3. Clean the chosen site with an alcohol-impregnated swab and allow to dry.
> 4. Pinch the skin.
> 5. Insert the needle into the skin at a 45° angle and release the pinched skin. Check that the needle is angled downwards into the subcutaneous tissue and not upwards into the superficial skin layer.
> 6. Tape the butterfly 'wings' using a transparent dressing.
> 7. Document the date and time of the procedure in the nursing notes.
> 8. Check the patency of the line before commencing an infusion.

How do I monitor central venous pressure?

Nicola Brooks

Central venous pressure (CVP) is the pressure in the right atrium of the heart (Mooney and Comerford, 2003). It is measured by inserting a central venous catheter into the right atrium and connecting it to a manometer. The indications for monitoring a patient's CVP (Mooney and Comerford, 2003) are:

- to monitor haemodynamic status in patients who are critically ill
- to monitor patients postoperatively
- to facilitate the diagnosis of cardiac failure
- administration of IV medication where the medication is an irritant when give by peripheral infusion (to monitor its effects on CVP)
- administration of large volumes of fluid (to monitor their effect on CVP in situations such as shock)
- administration of parenteral nutrition.

A 'normal' CVP reading can vary, so when you are recording a measurement it is important to ascertain what range the medical team would like readings to be maintained at. Research suggests that a simple manometer set gives a range of 3–12 cmH_2O, whereas with a transducer set the normal range is 0–8 mmHg. It is also important to take serial readings to establish a trend, so that abnormalities can be detected (Hatchett, 2000).

Taking a CVP measurement

The CVP measurement can be taken from either the mid-axilla (so that the baseline of the manometer set is in line with the right atrium) or the sternal notch. However, it is important to take readings from one position to ensure accuracy of the result. Readings taken for the sternal notch are about 5 cmH_2O lower than those taken from the mid-axilla.

Equipment required

- Infusion stand
- Manometer set
- Bag of fluid for readings (normally 0.9% sodium chloride)
- Spirit level

Procedure

1. Explain the procedure to the patient and gain his/her consent.
2. Gather equipment needed for the procedure.
3. Connect the manometer set to the infusion stand, and run the fluid through the infusion line. (Always seek advice if you are unsure of the procedure.)
4. Use the spirit level to make sure that the patient is level with the zero marker on the manometer set to ensure an accurate result.
5. Turn off the three-way tap to the patient. This will allow the manometer to fill slowly with fluid from the infusion bag. Do not overfill the chamber.
6. Turn off the three-way tap to the infusion fluid. This will cause the fluid in the manometer set to fall.
7. The reading can be taken when the level of fluid stops falling and settles to a rise and fall with the patient's respiration.
8. Record the CVP reading on the patient's observation chart and report any abnormalities to the medical team.
9. Turn off the three-way tap to the manometer and adjust the infusion rate as per prescription (to keep CVP line patent).
10. Document in the nursing notes where the reading has to be taken from (mid-axilla or sternal notch) to ensure accuracy of future readings.

What do I need to know about different wound dressings?
Nicola Brooks

There is a huge variety of wound dressings available today, with companies competing with each other to produce the ideal dressing.

Dressings are split into two categories: primary and secondary. A primary dressing is one that is in direct contact with the wound, and a secondary dressing is one that is superimposed over a primary dressing.

Factors to consider when selecting a dressing

- Ritualistic practice (is it something that has always been used?)
- Evidence-based practice
- Clinical experience
- Resources available (expense, availability)
- Patient preference (comfort)

- Where the wound is situated
- Size of the wound
- What will work for which type of wound?

Characteristics of the optimum wound dressing

The ideal dressing in wound care is one that provides optimal conditions for wound healing and prevents further damage to the surrounding areas. Turner (1985) identifies several characteristics of the optimum dressing – such a dressing would need to:

- maintain a high humidity between the wound and dressing (to promote a faster rate of epithelialisation)
- remove excess exudate and toxic compounds
- allow gaseous exchange
- provide thermal insulation at the wound surface
- be impermeable to wound bacteria
- be free from particles and wound contaminants
- allow removal without causing trauma at dressing change.

Types of wound dressing

The main types of wound dressing are:

- **Hydrocolloids:** These interact with wound exudate when in contact with the wound. They slowly absorb fluid to change the state of the dressing by forming a gel. This type of dressing can be used on infected wounds. The dressing should extend approximately 2 cm around the wound edge.

- **Hydrogels:** Used to deslough/debride wounds. When in contact with the wound they absorb exudate to provide a moist environment. These dressings are available as a flat sheet or gel, but require a secondary dressing to keep them in place.

- **Alginates:** Manufactured from seaweed. Form a gel when in contact with a wound. Suitable for use on exudating wounds.

- **Hydrofibres:** Used to deslough/debride wounds as a primary dressing for moderate to heavily exudating wounds. Available as a woven pad or ribbon of hydrocolloid fibres.

- **Foams:** Used for exudating flat or cavity wounds with differing absorbencies. Should not be used on dry wounds because of the risk of adherence.

- **Vapour-permeable films:** These are used to treat shallow wounds, or prophylactically to prevent pressure damage, or as a retention dressing.

They can be left in place for up to 7 days; however, care must be taken on removal to prevent trauma to fragile skin. The skin around the wound must be kept clean and dry.

- **Tulles:** An open-weave cotton dressing impregnated with paraffin, which requires frequent changes to prevent it drying out. They are difficult to remove if adherent, and become bedded in granulation tissue.

- **Iodine-based products:** These dressings contain a broad-spectrum antiseptic, although the effects of the dressing may be reduced by the presence of pus or exudate. They can cause sensitivity in some patients.

- **Silver-based products:** These dressings have antibacterial properties contained in a dressing or cream form. Side-effects have been reported with the long-term use of silver. The dressings can be used prophylactically as a dressing on line insertion sites, e.g. Hickman lines.

- **Wound manager bags:** These products are used to control exudate on high output wounds and protect the surrounding skin. Ideally they are used to monitor the yield of exudate from a wound. They can be left in place for a long period.

- **Larval therapy:** Larvae are not often a first-line choice of wound dressings. The sterile larvae of the common green bottle (*Lucilia sericate*) are used to debride the wound and remove bacteria. They are used and disposed of according to strict protocol, and ordered specifically for single patient use.

- **VAC therapy** Vacuum-assisted closure (VAC) therapy is used to apply negative pressure to a specialised dressing positioned in the wound cavity. Nursing staff may require extra training in the use of VAC pumps and equipment, to use them effectively. The dressing can be left in situ for a few days.

- **Paste bandages** These products consist of cotton bandages impregnated with a medical paste. Secondary dressings are required to secure them in place. Allergic reactions are common with this form of dressing. Paste bandages are often used in the treatment of thrombophlebitis.

When using any form of wound dressing, careful patient assessment is essential. It is advisable to use a wound assessment tool to ensure reliable and consistent documentation. Wounds should be reassessed regularly to evaluate the treatment given, as no single product is suitable for all wound types or all stages of healing. A flexible approach to the selection of wound care products is required to optimise the healing process.

What does an aseptic technique involve?

Nicola Brooks

Aseptic technique is a method of preventing microorganisms from reaching vulnerable sites (Briggs *et al*, 1996). It is the term used to describe the effort taken to keep the patient as free from hospital microorganisms as possible (Crows, 1989). Aseptic techniques are used to prevent contamination of wounds that could lead to infection, and is achieved by ensuring that only sterile equipment is used during invasive procedures.

Equipment required

- Sterile dressing pack
- Fluid for irrigation (if required)
- Appropriate dressing
- Hand hygiene preparation (according to local policy)
- Dressing trolley
- Scissors
- Tape
- Plastic apron

Procedure

1. Explain the procedure to the patient and gain his/her consent. Ensure patient comfort before the procedure.
2. Clean the dressing trolley with alcoholic preparation (according to local policy).
3. Place required equipment on the bottom shelf of the trolley.
4. Take all equipment to the patient's bedside, and put on plastic apron.
5. Loosen the dressing around the wound.
6. Wash your hands and apply bactericidal alcohol hand rub.
7. Check the sterility of all equipment – open the sterile field using only the corners of the paper.
8. Open all other sterile packs and tip contents onto the sterile field.
9. Wash your hands again and apply bactericidal alcohol hand rub.
10. Place your hand in the disposable bag (inside the dressing pack) to remove the used dressing. Invert the bag and stick onto the dressing trolley.
11. Put on sterile gloves, touching only the wrist end of the gloves.
12. Irrigate or clean the wound as necessary.
13. Change the dressing as required.
14. Dispose of all used equipment in the clinical waste after the procedure.

What are the principles of preparing patients for tests and investigations?

Penny Harrison

Bick (2000) suggests that the newly qualified nurse experiences a range of anxieties relating to the 'reality' of practice in the period of transition from student to registered nurse. Major foci of these anxieties include the nurse's perception of how much he/she does not know. This can be applied to the knowledge relating to the preparation of patients for tests and investigations. However, there is a wide range of help at hand. It is beyond the scope of this chapter and book to list every common test and investigation, and its related nursing care. This section aims to share some principles of preparing patients for a variety of tests and investigations, which can be used regardless of the specialty or type of healthcare setting the nurse finds him/herself in.

Useful references can be found at the end of the book. You could also develop your own small reference guide. I suggest that you have a hardbound notebook of A5 size. This is small enough to be carried in your uniform pocket. You can add information about tests and investigations in your area of practice as you participate in caring for a number of patients. You could also use this notebook for information gained from other chapters in this book, helping to build your own unique reference guide.

Activity break

❖ Identify an experienced nurse who works in the same area as you. Ask your colleague if they feel confident that they have the knowledge and skills relating to every test and investigation that patients may undergo? Ask them where they would go for further information if needed?

Reflection

❖ Did your colleague 'know all there is to know'? If not, does it surprise you that they do not necessarily know everything about every test or investigation that a patient can undergo?

❖ What skills did your colleague tell you about that they can utilise if they need to seek further information about tests and investigations?

Key principles of preparing patients for tests and investigations

Evans (2001) suggests that the expectations that newly qualified nurses have about their level of skills may reflect under-confidence and uncertainty. In my experience as a ward manager, newly qualified nurses are often a harsher judge of their abilities than experienced colleagues who are supporting them through the period of preceptorship.

The key to learning about the wide range of tests and investigations that patients undergo is to:

- Identify the common tests and investigations that take place in the current clinical setting – become familiar and confident with the 'everyday'. Do not worry about remembering details for every possible test and investigation.

- Know where to find further information and who you can ask for further advice or assistance – colleagues in the healthcare team prefer you to ask if you are unsure, and are usually keen to share their knowledge, expertise and experience.

- Participate actively in the care of the patient pre-test, during the test and post-test or investigation. Seeing the patient journey through tests and investigations helps you to remember the detail of care required.

- Reflect on how much you do know and are confident with – this will help you to identify gaps in your knowledge and clinical experience. Remember that you can make this into an action plan for completing the preceptorship programme, as well as using this evidence as part of your ongoing professional development to meet post-registration education and practice (PREP) requirements (NMC, 2004d).

Activity break

List the common tests that are undertaken for patients in your clinical setting. You might want to list them into groups as follows:

- Blood tests – haematology, biochemistry, microbiology, others
- Radiological tests – X-rays, computerised tomography (CT), magnetic resonance imaging (MRI), ultrasound, angiography
- Endoscopic tests – oesophagogastroduodenoscopy (OGD), sigmoidoscopy, colonoscopy
- Other tests, e.g. swallowing assessment by the speech and language therapist (SALT).

Reflection

Using your list as a basis for reflection, do you:

- Know what the tests/investigations are for, and what information about the patient's condition will be gained?
- What care the patient requires before the test?
- What care the patient requires during the test?
- What care the patient requires after the test?

Patient information

According to Evans (2001), patients typically request the following information before tests and investigations:

- Why do I need this test?
- How is it carried out?
- Where do I go for this test?
- How do I prepare for this test?
- How long will it take?
- When do I hear the results?
- What do the results mean?

Patient information is important not only for the sharing of information and communication with the patient, but also as part of the process of gaining consent. Additionally, it enables the patient to cope with the test or investigation: an informed patient is much more able to cooperate with the healthcare team during the test. Sufficient time spent preparing the patient for the test or investigation will be beneficial in terms of a speedy conclusion and satisfactory outcome for both the patient and the healthcare team (Walsh, 2003).

Activity break

- Familiarise yourself with local practice on the giving of information before tests and investigations.
- Ensure that you know where to find patient information leaflets on the tests and investigations that you are preparing patients for in your practice setting.

Reflection

- Reflect on how you and the healthcare team would give patients information about tests and investigations when:
    - The patient is confused.
    - The patient is blind or deaf.
    - The patient requires information in another language.

Tests, investigations and consent

An important part of preparing patients for tests and investigations is gaining their consent. Nurses undertake many aspects of care for patients on a daily basis, e.g. assisting with activities of daily living or observations. The *Code of Professional Conduct* (NMC, 2004a) states that the patient's consent and co-operation for care must be given. For many aspects of care, verbal consent is sufficient. For example, assisting the patient to wash and dress requires the nurse to gain verbal consent from the patient, but not formal written consent.

For more invasive tests and investigations, however, written consent is required. The Department of Health has issued guidance on consent (Department of Health, 2001b), with a set of standard consent forms introduced across the NHS in April 2002. In practice, the consent form is used in conjunction with the local consent policy. For example, local policy will usually require written consent for tests and investigations of an invasive nature, but not for less invasive procedures such as blood tests. The consent form requires the practitioner to give demographic information about the patient, list the test investigation or procedure to be carried out, and any particular risks that the patient may be exposed to. Emphasis is placed on the validity of consent, where correct completion of the consent form is the evidence of this, rather than a completed form that does not truly reflect the patient's consent to treatment or reflect true understanding of the benefits of the test, information to be gained and any potential risks or complications.

Activity break

- Familiarise yourself with your local trust's policy on consent.
- Ensure that you know where to find the consent forms in your practice setting.
- From your list of common tests and investigations that you previously compiled, note which require verbal consent and which require written consent. Discuss your ideas with a senior colleague to see if they agree.

Reflection

- Reflect on how you and the healthcare team would gain consent for tests and investigations from:
  - The patient who is confused.
  - The patient who has communication difficulties.
  - The patient who does not have English as a first language.
  - The patient in an emergency situation.

Pre-, peri- and post-investigation/test care

The specific pre-, peri- and post-care for all tests and investigations is beyond the scope of this section. However, the nurse needs to be familiar with some key principles before preparing patients for tests and investigations. Dougherty and Lister (2002) and Walsh (2003) have excellent chapters on the preparation of patients for tests and investigations, as well as details of specific care. Information from these texts can be summarised as:

- **Pre-test care** Communication, patient assessment, information giving, consent, sedation or anaesthesia, observations, specific blood tests.

- **Peri-test care** Communication, patient assessment, privacy and dignity, positioning and comfort, pain relief, observations, specific care.

✱ **Post-test care** Communication, patient assessment, information giving, recovery from sedation (or anaethesia), positioning and comfort, pain relief, observations, specific care, follow-up care.

> ### Activity break
> ❖ As an example, familiarise yourself with the care required for a patient undergoing an oesophagogastroduodenoscopy (OGD).
> ❖ Using the checklists above, identify the care required for a patient undergoing an OGD in your practice setting.
> ❖ If you are not sure about the specific care involved, identify where you would go to seek further advice, help and information.
>
> ### Reflection
> ❖ Reflect on:
>   - the aspects of care that you were familiar with
>   - the aspects of care that you were not familiar with
>   - the sources of help you could utilise.
> ❖ Using the information in this section, reflect on how you can continue to acquire knowledge and skills to nurse patients in your practice setting for a range of tests and investigations.

Tests, investigations and record keeping

The NMC (2004a) requires practitioners to maintain accurate, chronological records for all aspects of patient care. Effective record keeping is a key tool in maintaining high standards of professional practice. Detailed guidance is provided by the NMC (2004e). Record keeping for tests and investigations may involve recording information about aspects of the care and management of the patient requiring observations, fluid balance management, as well as how well the test or investigation was tolerated and the recovery process.

Additional information, which it is equally important to record, is details of communications between the patient, his/her family or carers and the multiprofessional team. Reflection on the nature of the meeting and details of how a patient received or appeared to receive information is a unique part of the nurse's role. The records assist the nurse in coordinating care across the team in a cooperative and constructive manner (NMC, 2004a).

A key part of record keeping in relation to patient safety during tests and investigations is correct labelling of specimens. Many specimens will be sent for review and/or reporting by technical staff in the laboratories. Inaccurate labelling of specimens may not only delay further pathological reporting, but also dangerous if the specimen becomes mixed with other patient specimens. Information relating to the patient's condition may be diagnosed incorrectly, treatment delayed or unnecessary treatment commenced. Thus safe handling of specimens is as important as other aspects of record keeping.

Activity break

* As an example, familiarise yourself with the care required for a patient undergoing oesophagogastroduodenoscopy (OGD).
* Identify the patient records and charts required for OGD in your practice setting.
* Identify the process for labelling specimens taken from the patient undergoing OGD in your practice setting.

Reflection

* Reflect on the wide range of records that you would use to maintain accurate patient records for this test/investigation. Did your list include any of the following:
  * medical notes and X-rays?
  * consent form?
  * results from blood tests?
  * admission documentation, nursing notes?
  * discharge documentation, letter to the GP?
* Reflect on the range of documentation used. Was there scope for duplication or omission of information?
* Reflect on the process used to label specimens. Is there any risk of error in this process. What is the role of the nurse in minimising such risk?

Drug administration specific to tests and investigations

The NMC requires practitioners to administer medications to patients in a safe manner (NMC, 2004c; see chapter on drug administration). Drugs required for tests and investigations may include sedatives before the test, analgesics during the test or prophylactic antibiotics to prevent or reduce the risk of infection following the test.

Activity break

* As an example, familiarise yourself with the care required for a patient undergoing oesophagogastroduodenoscopy (OGD).
* Identify the drugs required for a patient undergoing OGD in your practice setting.

Reflection

* Reflect on your knowledge of the drugs used for the patient undergoing OGD. Were you familiar with:
  * the drugs?
  * the rationale for their use?
  * the potential side-effects?
  * any drugs used for a potential emergency during the OGD?

Tests and investigations form a key part of care for all patients. The nurse is well placed to coordinate care for patients requiring tests and investigations across the healthcare team (Alexander *et al*, 2000; NMC, 2004a; Walsh, 2003). It is unrealistic to expect the nurse to be an expert on all tests and investigations. However, the principles of this key part of health care apply across all healthcare settings. Competence and confidence in using these principles will assist the nurse in ensuring that the patient receives the best standard of care possible while undergoing a wide range of tests and investigations.

How can I promote continence?

Penny Tremayne

There are few things that erode a person's self-esteem and dignity more than incontinence. Many people who suffer from incontinence are often too embarrassed to seek help, even from their GP or practice nurse, and consequently 'suffer in silence'. It is important that the nurse takes a positive approach to the promotion of continence and, if necessary, the management of incontinence. Good communication and social skills are required if the nurse is to build up the essential nurse–patient relationship that is crucial in this situation.

Key points

- Initial and ongoing assessment. Identify normal pattern and type of incontinence – is it stress, urge, overflow or functional?

- Availability of facilities and aids, e.g. bedpan, commode, wheelchair, raised toilet seats, a call bell that is within reach and its use understood.

- Recognition of special needs. This includes patients who have an urgency and frequency, those who are confused or have an altered level of awareness, those who are prone to hypotension (Dowse and MacKender, 2000), as well as those with impaired manual dexterity.

- An agreed continence regimen that places the patient at the centre, with a team of nurses who have the motivation to apply the regimen, which may include:
  - gradually lengthening the time between voiding (Dowse and MacKender, 2000)
  - timed voiding
  - prompted voiding.

- Maintenance of an accurate, ongoing continence chart.

- Other containment methods – these commonly include:

- pads and pants – ensure that they are fitted correctly and that the pad is appropriate (is it for slight leaking, heavy leakage, day or overnight use?)
- sheaths – especially in men – ensure that the appropriate size is used and that the sheath is applied according to the manufacturer's guidelines
- catheterisation.

⌘ Referral to continence advisor.

⌘ Pelvic floor exercises.

⌘ Referral to physiotherapy and occupational therapy.

⌘ Intermittent self-catheterisation.

⌘ Maintenance of dignity, respect and privacy.

What are the most common signs and symptoms of a urinary tract infection?

Penny Tremayne

⌘ Patients usually only display the signs and symptoms of a urinary tract infection once the bacteria have invaded the bladder mucosa and, as a consequence, caused inflammation (Godfrey and Evans, 2001).

⌘ Frequency in passing small amounts of urine.

⌘ Pain on micturition; this has been described as 'like passing glass'.

⌘ Lower lumbar pain (from the kidneys).

⌘ Urine may smell offensive (fishy), appear cloudy and may even be slightly bloodstained or contain mucus or debris.

⌘ Elderly patients may become confused.

⌘ Some patients with urinary tract infection may not display or report any of these signs or symptoms, and therefore urinalysis should be performed and the results recorded on an ongoing basis.

What should I do if I suspect that a patient has a urinary tract infection?

⌘ If the urine is obviously infected, obtain a specimen as soon as possible.
⌘ If you are unsure whether the urine is infected, perform a urinalysis. If blood, protein, nitrates or leucocyctes are present, obtain a clean specimen for culture and microscopy (Colley, 1998).

- ⌘ Record and monitor temperature and pulse rate at least 4-hourly
- ⌘ Record and monitor an accurate fluid balance chart.
- ⌘ Inform medical staff.
- ⌘ Encourage a fluid intake of at least 1.5 litres daily if appropriate (Addison, 1999).

What do I need to know about pressure ulcers?
Penny Tremayne

Arguably, the development of a pressure ulcer within the healthcare setting can be seen as an indicator of the quality of nursing care that a patient is receiving. Costs are significant, not only financially to the NHS, but also emotionally and physically to the patient.

How do I identify whether a patient is at risk of developing a pressure ulcer?

The first step in preventing pressure ulcers is to undertake a pressure ulcer risk assessment. This should be seen as a dynamic tool and should serve as an aide-mémoire only, and not replace clinical judgment (Royal College of Nursing, 2001).

Assessment should include a full examination of every patient's skin integrity over all the bony prominences: back of the head, temporal region of the skull, ear, shoulders, elbows, hip, thigh, leg, buttocks, rib cage, sacrum, knees, heels and toes. The Royal College of Nursing (2001) also highlights the 'ischial tuberosities, parts of body affected by anti-embolic stockings (ensure correctly measured for and fitted correctly), parts of the body affected where pressure, friction and shear are exerted in the course of daily activities, parts of the body where there is external force from clothing or equipment'. Nasal cannuale, for example, can cause possible breakdown of skin integrity on the bridge of the nose, inside the nose, the cheeks, and the ear (Royal College of Nursing, 2001).

Too often in documentation the phrase 'skin intact' is written, and yet the skin has not been fully inspected. Always ensure accuracy when writing about skin integrity.

Which patients are most at risk of developing a pressure ulcer?

The key is not to make assumptions about who is at risk and who is not at risk of developing a pressure ulcer. The Royal College of Nursing (2001) identifies some intrinsic risk factors that should prompt you into action (*Box 3.3*).

What should I do if a patient is at risk of developing a pressure ulcer?

Whatever the merits of any assessment scale, it will be of no use unless you act on the results of the assessment (Cook *et al*, 1999; Reed *et al*, 2001). If the patient is at risk of developing a pressure ulcer, then follow the stages of the

> **Box 3.3**
> **Risk factors associated with pressure ulcer development**
>
> - Immobile/reduced mobility
> - Sensory impairment
> - Acute illness
> - Reduced level of consciousness
> - Extremes of age (up to 65 years, or less than 5 years)
> - Previous history of damage
> - Vascular disease
> - Severe chronic/terminal illness
> - Malnutrition
> - Dehydration
> - Medication
> - Moisture

nursing process, ensure that there is a realistic, accurate and individualised care plan agreed and that this is implemented and evaluated accordingly.

The care plan will include a goal – what is to be achieved. This can be immediate, but is more usually medium term or even ongoing, but must include a review/goal date. So, for example, a generic ongoing goal for a patient at risk of developing pressure ulcers might be:

> 'Mr / Mrs / Ms / Miss ………………… *will not develop any pressure ulcers as a consequence of being in the healthcare setting – Review: Every Sunday*'

A more specific goal for a patient who has developed a pressure ulcer might read:

> 'Mr / Mrs / Ms / Miss…………………..*grade 3 pressure ulcer will show signs of healing and be …………mm reduced in width, …………mm reduced in length, and ………..mm reduced in depth by date……………………*

Photographic evidence or a measurement template may also be useful here. Always ensure that the patient's consent is obtained. Include a ruler in the photograph so that accurate measurements can be made.

The care plan should be evidence based and can include care such as that outlined below (this list is not exhaustive):

- Repositioning the patient according to individualised need, usually every 2 or 3 hours, to prevent damage to the skin and underlying structures (Royal College of Nursing, 2001).

- Adoption of an appropriate moving and handling procedure to reduce damage to the skin from shearing and friction, applying local protocol/policy for patient handling.

⌘ A pressure-reducing/relieving mattress should be selected according to the patient's condition, comfort and assessment of risk. There are a number of mattresses available:

- standard foam
- higher specification pressure-reducing foam
- non-dynamic (static) pressure-relieving overlays
- dynamic pressure-relieving (alternating inflation and deflation of cells)
- alternating inflation overlays (one layer of air cells)
- replacement (double layer of alternating air cells)
- low air-loss (air is gradually lost through tiny holes, combined with continuous inflation)
- air-fluidised bead beds
- specialist support systems

(Guy, 2004)

Low air-loss and static air mattresses have been found to be effective in the critical care setting, and alternating-pressure air mattresses have been found to be effective in the elderly, medical, orthopaedic as well as the critical care setting (Gebhardt, 2002).

⌘ A pressure-redistributing cushion can be used as long as good posture is facilitated and the cushion does not interfere with mobilisation. Evidence to support the use of such cushions is limited (Clarke, 2002; Gebhardt, 2002), and the National Institute for Clinical Excellence (2001) recommends that patients who are considered to be acutely at risk of developing pressure ulcers should be restricted to sitting in a chair for less than 2 hours.

⌘ Maintain or promote a balanced diet and adequate hydration – to minimise the patient's vulnerability to pressure as well as maintain elasticity of the tissues.

⌘ Make sure that the skin is clean, dry and well moisturised – cleanse skin as soon as possible after soiling, use mild detergents in conjunction with warm water to prevent drying and irritation, and apply moisturiser to any dry skin (Agency for Health Care Policy and Prevention, 1992). There are also some non-water-based foams available, which clean and moisten the skin.

⌘ If the patient requires a dressing for a pressure ulcer, as a registered nurse you should select one that is clinically effective. Consider the manufacturer's recommendations and a wound care formulary (Grayless *et al*, 2002). Evaluation – a judgment on the effectiveness of the delivery of care – should be made if the patient' condition improves or deteriorates, or on the review/goal date. Thus the previous stages, such as assessment and planning, might have to be revisited. Phrases that should be avoided are:

'Turned regularly' – Your birthday is regular: once a year. Are you turning the patient annually?

'Turned 2 hourly' – A description of what you are doing, but no clinical judgment on the state of the skin.

'Pressure sore dressing changed according to care plan' – What does the pressure ulcer look like? Is there any exudate? If so, is it a mild, moderate or heavy exudate? Is the pressure ulcer epithelialising, granulating, sloughy, necrotic, infected or fungating/malodorous? It may be useful to compare the appearance with the photograph or original measurement template.

⌘ Don't forget that most trusts have a tissue viability specialist nurse to whom you can refer directly.

If a patient develops, or is admitted or transferred, to your ward with a pressure ulcer, an incident form should be completed. This enables the trust to monitor the occurrence of pressure ulcers.

How do I help my patients meet their nutritional needs?
Penny Tremayne

It is well known that patients in the healthcare setting are often malnourished (Bond, 1997). It is essential that patients are adequately nourished. Malnutrition can increase physical and psychological stress as well as affecting almost every body system (Horan and Coad, 2000).

As a registered nurse, you are ultimately responsible for ensuring that patients' nutritional needs are met. At times there can be a tendency to focus on the more technical aspects of feeding, such as parenteral and enteral feeding methods.

How should I perceive mealtimes?

Mealtimes should have a high priority. It is important that patients who are acutely ill have appropriate nutritional input. Patients who are recovering perceive mealtimes as an important social event in the day, as well as providing appropriate constituents for body repair. As a registered nurse, you should try to facilitate an environment that is conducive to eating, e.g. reduce disturbances (Anderson, 2000) and try to make sure that patients have the opportunity to use a commode before mealtimes. Communicate effectively with catering, nursing and domestic staff (Horan and Coad, 2000). Make sure you act as a role model: demonstrate the importance of nutritional monitoring by getting involved, observing, and monitoring and recording whether patients are eating or being given the opportunity to eat. Some patients might not eat much because they are anxious or worried, so take the opportunity to talk to your patients and use the meal as a prompt to ask them how they feel.

How can I recognise if a patient is at risk of being malnourished?

Assessment of nutritional status is pivotal and should include the following:

- Identification of the patient's 'norm'; too often, phrases such as 'eats well' or 'no problems' are included in admission details. Explore further. What food does the patient eat? What food does he/she prefer? Is he/she physically able to shop? Can the patient afford the food or the fuel to cook the food? Is he/she physically able to cook? What amount of food does the patient normally eat?

- Identification of the patient's ability on admission and on an ongoing basis. Is the patient able to eat, e.g. does he/she have a gag/swallowing reflex? Is the patient able to feed him/herself? Does the patient have any specialist or therapeutic dietary needs?

- Undertake an ongoing nutritional risk assessment. This can indicate whether a patient is at no risk, moderate risk, high risk or very high risk of malnourishment (McLaren *et al*, 1997). Ensure that if the patient is at any risk, then an individualised care plan is agreed, implemented and evaluated.

- Consider weighing the patient once or twice weekly (as the patient's condition dictates).

- Observe the patient's general condition and bodily appearance.

What can I do if a patient is not eating very much?

- Try to identify the cause. Is it related to a sore mouth, coated tongue, nausea, vomiting, abdominal discomfort, constipation, diarrhoea or pain?

- Encourage the patient's family to bring in food that the patient likes and to actively participate in the nutritional care of the patient.

- Maintain an accurate food chart. Avoid writing phrases such as 'fish – all' – what does this mean? There is a difference between a whole cod and a sardine. Specify the amount eaten, whether it is a teaspoonful or a tablespoonful.

- Offer nutritional supplements as appropriate, e.g. if no food is being taken, offer a milk-based or nutrient-rich soup or pudding as a food substitute; ensure that these are given at the appropriate time and recorded (McLaren *et al*, 1997).

- For other supplements and dietary advice, request appropriate referral and/or prescription. Some supplements can be potentially harmful as they have high levels of nutrients (Barton *et al*, 2000, Green, 2000). Patients unable to be adequately nourished by mouth may receive enteral feeding via a nasogastric tube (often fine-bore) or percutaneous endoscopic gastrostomy.

What principles do practical nursing skills involve?

Personal notes and contacts

Chapter 4

How do I discharge patients or refer them to other services?

Tracey Kemmett

- ❖ How do I refer patients to the community services?
- ❖ How do I refer patients to the multidisciplinary team?
- ❖ How do I refer patients to specialist nurses?

How do I refer patients to the community services?

General principles when referring or discharging patients

Each service will have a specific referral form that will need to be completed. Find out where these forms are located, what information is required and where they need to be sent once they are completed. Ensure that the referral is recorded in the patient's documentation, including the date, whom the referral has been sent to, and your signature and designation.

When should I refer patients to the community services?

This depends on the patient's health needs. If the patient has relatively simple requirements, such as suture removal, the referral can be carried out the day before discharge during the normal working week (Monday to Friday). If the patient is being discharged at a weekend or beginning of a bank holiday period, the service may be limited, so ensure that the referral is carried out with at least one working day's notice. If in doubt, contact those who will be providing the care and ask for advice.

If the patient's needs are complex or particularly specialised, early referral to the community services is essential. Continuing health care is where health needs are beyond that which is normally expected, e.g. visits from a district nurse three times a week.

The assessment, which is usually performed by a registered nurse, will start the process for obtaining specialist equipment or particular care such as 24-hour home nursing. This documentation should ask key questions that identify health needs or requirements for assessment by the multidisciplinary team.

More complex care may require input from social services as well as the health services. Contacting all who need to be involved as early as possible will reduce the chance of finding something that has not been addressed on the day of discharge, which could result in a delay in the patient's discharge.

Why refer patients to the community services?

An admission to hospital may identify or create the need for additional care support once the patient returns home. An assessment carried out on a patient's admission to hospital may reveal that the patient is not coping in their current home environment, or that the effects of operative intervention or illness will affect their ability to achieve a quality of life safely. So, what would that patient need? Image how the patient would cope if you were to send them home the next day. Assessing the full picture is vital; think about the everyday activities that the patient may need assistance with and who could provide this.

Appropriate referral depends on accurate needs assessment of the patient and knowledge of the systems and services available locally. If sutures need removing, a practice nurse can do this, or if the patient is unable to get to the GP, then a visit from a district nurse will need to be arranged. If the patient has complex needs that require frequent nursing intervention, the district nurse may wish to visit and assess the patient before discharge.

Within health care there is always some type of waiting involved and referrals are no exception. A referral made in hospital may require follow-up in the community. In the case of a patient needing podiatry (chiropody) care, the referral would be sent out to the community if the patient has been discharged from hospital before being assessed.

How do I refer patients to the community services?

Hospitals will have a list of GP surgeries to be contacted for services such as district nurses, health visitors, practice nurses and other specialist nurses within the community. If your hospital has a discharge coordinator, then they will also have a contact list. If all else fails, look up the patient's GP in the phone directory, call them and seek advice about the services provided by that practice. Having a named person to contact always gets better results.

Complete the appropriate community referral form. Ensure that it adheres to all the guidelines relating to completion of patient documentation. Document in the patient's records that the referral has been made and the date of referral. Make sure the following details are included in the referral form:

- name and address
- date of birth
- GP's name and address
- medical history – does the patient have a long-term illness such as diabetes or rheumatoid arthritis?
- any medication that the patient has been prescribed
- clear and concise reason for the referral
- date and sign the form.

Helping others to prioritise referrals

If you add URGENT to all community referrals without an explanation, then the person receiving the referral will have no way of prioritising their work. If the referral is urgent, then make that clear on the referral form and add reasons why this is so. An additional telephone call to the person in question will enable you to highlight the urgent needs of this particular patient. That person will also be happy to answer any queries you may have with regard to referrals – just pick up the phone and ask. Don't forget to inform patients of the approximate time interval, e.g. days, weeks or months, before they can expect to be contacted by the referred service.

How do I refer patients to the multidisciplinary team?

General principles when referring or discharging patients

Each service will have a specific referral form that will need to be completed. Find out where these forms are located, what information is required and where they need to be sent once they are completed. Ensure that the referral is recorded in the patient's documentation, including the date, whom the referral has been sent to and your signature and designation.

The multidisciplinary team can include physiotherapists, occupational therapists, dietitian, podiatrist, speech therapist, counsellor and many others.

When and why should I refer patients to the multidisciplinary team?

This will depend on the assessed needs of the patient. As a nurse, you will assess, plan and deliver the nursing care required by the patient, but will need to refer the patient to other members of the multidisciplinary team for either advice or specific treatment. It is when the patient requires more than just nursing care that a referral will be needed. In all cases it is better to make a referral straight away to maximise the recovery of the patient.

So, what does the multidisciplinary team do?

- **Physiotherapists** concentrate on strength and movement of the body. They can help patients to adapt to certain illnesses or operative procedures. They plan rehabilitation programmes, aiming to enhance patients' recovery. If walking aids are likely to be required following an operation, a referral preoperatively would be appropriate.

- **Occupational therapists** work in conjunction with physiotherapists to enhance a patient's rehabilitation. Their work may involve making support splints to immobilise a joint, assessing the need for dressing aids or aids to everyday activities such as opening a jar or getting in the bath. They may also work with patients, helping them to find ways of conserving their energy and strength, e.g. patients with dypsnoea.

- **Dietitians** assess the nutritional status of patients and plan a diet to ensure that all their nutritional requirements are met. This may include supplements, nasogastric feeding or a weight loss diet. A patient with a poor dietary intake or a patient who has been newly diagnosed with diabetes will require a referral to the dietitian.

- **Podiatrists** specialise in feet and gait analysis, and work in hospitals and the community. If you are not sure of their input, contact the hospital department for advice, or ask one to visit your ward area and run a teaching session about their role. Cutting a patient's toenails can be a nurse's role *only* when you have been trained how to do this: if not, a referral if required.

- **Speech therapists** would be needed whenever a patient has difficulty in producing words or sounds, e.g. following trauma, maxillary surgery or a stroke, or for swallowing assessment for patients with dysphagia.

How do I refer patients to the multidisciplinary team?
In most wards, regular meetings take place between the nursing staff and members of the multidisciplinary team. Discussions are carried out as to which patients on the ward may require referral or assessment. If these meetings do not occur or if the referral is urgent, follow the referral system identified in the previous section. Once a member of the multidisciplinary team is seeing a patient, he/she will ensure that a referral is carried out if community involvement is required following discharge.

How do I refer patients to specialist nurses?

General principles when referring or discharging patients

Each service will have a specific referral form that will need to be completed. Find out where these forms are located, what information is required and where they need to be sent once they are completed. Ensure that the referral is recorded in the patient's documentation, including the date, whom the referral has been sent to and your signature and designation.

Specialist nurses have practical and theoretical knowledge within a specific area of practice. Sometimes this is an area of traditional nursing practice, such as stoma care, or it may be an area more traditionally associated with medical practice, such as pain. The variety and number of specialist nurses in your area will depend on the size of your hospital and the specialties in it. Specialist nurses commonly cover the following areas: asthma, diabetes, tissue viability, infection control, pain, palliative care, sports medicine, rehabilitation, operating departments and specialist outpatient clinics, such as infertility, surgical reconstructions and many more. Make a point of finding out which specialist nurses are available in your area of work.

When, why and how do I refer patients to specialist nurses?
Consult your local guidelines and policies; there may be a strategy written by the specialist nurse regarding what action to take and when to refer. A common

system is to have a link nurse on each ward or unit who has a direct link to the specialist lead. The link nurse can then hold regular teaching sessions, enabling the transfer of up-to-date information from the specialist lead to the ward staff or departmental staff. If such a link system operates within your hospital, find out who the link nurses are, how to contact them and their specific role.

To ensure that patients receive the treatment and care they require, as a general rule you should acknowledge your limitations and be aware of where additional experience or expertise lays. If it is beyond your competence and confidence, consult a more experienced nurse initially for advice. Discuss with the link nurse and, if necessary, the nurse specialist. Don't forget that this may be a unit or trust resource and will not necessarily be located on your ward. If a link nurse is not available or is unable to help you, the hospital will have a list of contact numbers to enable you to refer the patient to the specialist nurse. It may be that the medical consultant has advised you to involve the specialist nurse, so you do not have to make that decision.

As with all referrals, always be clear and concise with your information. Ask yourself why you are seeking their input, document the referral in the patient's records and never be afraid to ask for advice. Do not try to cope if you are not sure what to do – other professionals or specialists are there to help you provide the best care for your patient. Other professionals will not only be happy to answer any questions you have, but will also pass on some valuable knowledge to you in the process.

How do I discharge patients or refer them to other services?

Personal notes and contacts

Chapter 5

What are the principles of patient medication?

Annie Law

- What is the nurse's role in drug administration?
- What legislation governs medications and are there other national documents that guide us in this practice?
- How do drugs work?
- What are the principles of safe practice for administering medications?
- What do I need to know about drug calculations?
- What are the routes of drug administration?
- What are the ethical issues in drug administration?
- How can I avoid drug errors?
- What are the alternative and new initiatives in drug administration?

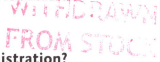

What is the nurse's role in drug administration?

The most frequent clinical intervention that registered nurses perform in the NHS today is drug administration. This area of practice is also the most frequent cause of anxiety in newly registered nurses. The complexity of drug regimens has increased with the continuous stream of new and novel drugs and patients receiving multiple drug therapy. This in turn increases the risk of adverse reactions and errors (Cavell, 2000).

To ensure safe and effective drug administration you need to maintain your knowledge of drugs at a high level and constantly update that knowledge. This chapter aims to provide you with the minimum knowledge you need in order to be a safe practitioner in drug administration. It is not the intention to cover all the common medications as there are sufficient sources available in all clinical areas for reference purposes.

To be able to administer drugs safely, a nurse needs to have sufficient knowledge in the following areas:

- Legislation related to drug therapy
- Pharmacology
- Principles of safe practice
- Drug calculations
- Routes of drug administration
- Ethical issues in drug administration
- Management of drug errors
- Alternative and new initiatives: self-administration; patient group directions; nurse prescribing.

What legislation governs medications and are there other national documents that guide us in this practice?

Legal and professional frameworks

Two key pieces of legislation govern the use of drugs:

- The Medicines Act 1968
- The Misuse of Drugs Act 1971.

Although these are somewhat dated, there have been statutory instruments (secondary legislation) to supplement these Acts as changes occur.

Medicines Act 1968

This Act controls the manufacture and distribution of medicines, i.e. who can lawfully supply and be in possession of medicines, and how medicines are packaged and labelled. The Act classifies drugs into three categories:

1. **Prescription-only medicines (POM):** Drugs that may only be supplied and administered to a patient on the instruction of an appropriate practitioner.
2. **Pharmacy-only medicines:** Drugs that can be purchased from a chemist shop only if the sale is supervised by a pharmacist.
3. **General sales list:** Drugs that do not need a prescription or supervision of a pharmacist – basically anything that you can buy in your local supermarket.

Misuse of Drugs Act 1971

This replaced the previous Dangerous Drugs Act, and controls the import, export, production, supply and possession of drugs of abuse. Changes in the legal status of some drugs have led to the Misuse of Drugs (Safe Custody) Regulations 1973 and the Misuse of Drugs Regulations 1985. These identify five separate schedules of controlled drugs, which you need to be familiar with as your responsibilities in terms of storage, checking and disposal relate to the different schedules.

Nursing implications

- Any discrepancies in the stock balance of controlled drugs may result in the police becoming involved. It is therefore vital that you familiarise yourself with local policies related to controlled drugs. You must know:
  - The correct storage of these drugs
  - The scrupulous checking required when administering these drugs to a patient and the stock balance each day
  - The disposal mechanisms
  - Record keeping.

Nurse Prescribing Act 1992

This piece of legislation reached the statute books directly as a result of the need for the law to catch up with the demands of the NHS (Shepherd, 2002c); this will be referred to again later in the chapter.

Nursing & Midwifery Council (NMC) Guidelines for the Administration of Medicines (NMC, 2004c)

These guidelines were produced by the professional regulatory body for nurses and midwives to provide guidance on the principles of safe drug administration. They will be discussed in more depth later in this chapter.

European Union (EU) directive

EU directive 92/27/EEC places a responsibility on each member of the EU to provide patients with information leaflets for each medicine dispensed. This became law in 1999.

> **Nursing implication**
>
> ❖ If you are teaching patients how to take their medication before leaving hospital or in their own homes, patient information leaflets provide a useful information source for you and your patient. You should ensure that the patient or their carer is aware of this information, which they can refer to if necessary when you are not there.

National Institute for Clinical Effectiveness (NICE)

NICE was set up by the Government in 1999, and although its role is to advise on best practice related to diagnostic techniques, medical devices, therapeutic interventions, as well as drug prescribing practices, its agenda has been dominated by the last category.

> **Nursing implication**
>
> ❖ You should keep yourself up to date with any new guidelines that NICE produce related to the prescribing of drugs for particular conditions. These guidelines can be found on the website for NICE at **www.nice.org.uk**

National Service Frameworks

These frameworks have been produced by expert groups working with the Government to provide guidance to clinicians and health service managers on best practice in terms of service provision, e.g. cancer, heart disease, mental health and older people. They contain guidance on specific drug therapy.

> **Nursing implication**
>
> ❖ Maintaining your knowledge of any frameworks connected with your specialty will not only help you to understand any recommendations for particular drugs, but also to understand why services may change and the impact that these changes may have on nursing. The National Service Frameworks can be viewed and downloaded from the Department of Health website **www.dh.gov.uk/Home/fs/en**

Other government documents

The Department of Health (Department of Health) published a report in 2000 entitled *An Organisation with a Memory* (Department of Health, 2000a). This report made two recommendations specific to medicines:

1. To decrease to 0 the number of patients dying or being paralysed by maladministered spinal injections.

2. To cut by 40% the number of serious errors in the use of prescribed drugs by 2004.

The Audit Commission has produced two documents concerned with medicines management, and made recommendations for cost savings, including promoting self-medication for most patients in hospital (Audit Commission, 2001, 2002).

> **Nursing implication**
>
> ❖ Keeping abreast of new reports from these bodies will help you to improve practice, maintain patient safety and avoid common errors. Audit Commission reports can be obtained from the websites **www.dh.gov.uk/Home/fs/en** and **www.audit-commission.gov.uk**

How do drugs work?

The use of drugs to treat ailments is not new; for thousands of years, extracts from plants and animals have been used to treat many illnesses and some are still used today, e.g. morphine, salicylates, digitalis (Goodinson, 1986a).

As a nurse, you need to have a basic understanding of how drugs reach their target cells and how they work, in order to understand the impact that normal

physiological processes and disease have on drug metabolism and excretion.
This section will cover the following aspects of pharmacology:

- drug distribution
- mechanism of drug action
- metabolism
- excretion
- adverse reactions.

Drug distribution

Once a drug enters the circulation, a proportion of it binds to plasma proteins, e.g. albumin – some to specific carrier proteins, and some to erythrocytes and other proteins – but it is only the proportion of drug that remains free in the plasma that reaches its target cells. As the free drug in the plasma leaves the circulation, the proportion of the drug that is bound to plasma proteins is released into the plasma.

This works fine if we only take one drug at a time, but many drugs compete for binding sites on the plasma proteins and literally knock each other off. This increases the amount of free drug in the plasma, resulting in the drug reaching its target cells sooner and therefore exerting a quicker effect, which in some cases can have serious consequences (Goodinson, 1986a; *Nursing Times*, 1994a; Shepherd, 2002a).

Examples

❖ Warfarin is displaced by tolbutamide, leading to an increased risk of haemorrhage.

❖ Tolbutamide is displaced by salicylates, leading to an increased risk of hypoglycaemia.

Drugs are either water or fat soluble. Those that are fat soluble, e.g. diazepam, are more widely distributed in the body and are able to cross the blood-brain barrier.

Clinical relevance

❖ Any change in the body due to the effects of disease can alter drug distribution and therefore the effect of the drug. For example, gentamicin is extremely water soluble; if there is fluid accumulation, such as ascites, the distribution and hence the effect of gentamicin is altered.

(John and Stevenson, 1995)

Mechanism of drug action

After the drug has travelled in the circulation to its target cells, how does it work? Drugs exert their effects in the body in several ways:

- They may replace missing substances – in vitamin deficiency, diabetes mellitus and hypothyroidism, for example.

- They may interfere with cell function by either stimulating or reducing the normal activity of messengers from one part of the body to another.

- They act against invading organisms or abnormal cells either by inhibiting multiplication of the organism or by killing it directly, e.g. antibiotics, antiviral and antifungal drugs (*Nursing Times*, 1994a).

Drug action occurs at the cell membrane level, and drugs are categorised as specific or non-specific.

Specific drugs

Specific drugs are drugs that attach to specific receptors on the surface of the cell membrane (Goodinson, 1986a).

Receptors

It is known that hormones and neurotransmitters exert their physiological effects, and drugs their pharmacological effects, by attaching to specific receptors on the cell membrane of the cells they are designed to target. This contact triggers events that result in the desired activity. When making contact with receptors, hormones, neurotransmitters and drugs can act as:

- **Agonists**
  These cause an observable response when they bind to a specific receptor on the cell membrane.

- **Partial agonists**
  These produce a limited response when they bind to a specific receptor, but at the same time prevent the actions of full agonists.

- **Antagonists**
  These do not produce a response when they bind to a specific receptor; instead they prevent the action of agonists.

Once a drug has bound to its specific receptor, there is often an increase in the concentration of an intracellular substance before the response occurs; this substance is known as a second messenger (Goodinson, 1986a; Shepherd, 2002a).

Examples of specific drugs

- Adrenaline is a beta-receptor agonist: it stimulates cardiac beta-receptors, causing an increase in heart rate.

- Fentanyl and diamorphine are opioid agonists: they mimic the body's own opioid neurotransmitters (endorphins) and produce their analgesic effect by activating the opioid receptors.

- Atenolol is a beta-receptor antagonist: it blocks cardiac beta-receptors, causing a decrease in heart rate.

- Prazocin and doxazocin block the action of alpha-adrenergic receptors in blood vessels, causing vasodilatation and thereby reducing blood pressure.

(John and Stevenson, 1995; Shepherd, 2002a)

Many drugs are not specific to one receptor and will act at more than one site or subset of receptors; this explains the known side-effects of some drugs.

Examples of specific drugs that act at more than one site

- Amitriptyline, a tricyclic antidepressant, blocks both the cholinergic and histamine receptors, causing the side-effects of dry mouth, blurred vision, constipation and drowsiness.

- Beta-blockers can attach to both the $beta_1$-receptors in the heart and $beta_2$-receptors in the lungs, the latter causing the side-effect of broncho-constriction. These drugs should therefore be avoided in asthmatics.

(John and Stevenson, 1995)

Some drugs compete with each other for receptor sites, or they may potentiate each's stimulating effect on the body.

Example
- If naloxone is given to a patient receiving morphine, the effects of morphine are reversed as naloxone knocks the morphine off its receptor.

(*Nursing Times*, 1994a; Shepherd, 2002a).

Non-specific drugs

Non-specific drug action is not mediated by receptors, but is dependent on other factors, such as:

- enzyme inhibition
- enzyme activation
- inhibition of cellular transport processes
- physico-chemical properties of the drug
- inhibition of biochemical processes (Goodinson, 1986a).

Examples of non-specific drugs

- Enalapril, ramipril and lisinopril are used in heart failure and hypertension: they act by inhibiting angiotensin-converting enzyme.

- Streptokinase and alteplase (fibrinolytic agents) activate plasminogen to form plasmin, which breaks down thrombi.

- Digoxin inhibits the sodium/potassium pump in the heart. Amlodipine, nifedipine and diltiazem (calcium-channel blockers) reduce smooth muscle contraction by blocking the calcium channels, resulting in relaxation of arteriolar smooth muscle. Lansoprazole, a proton pump inhibitor, inhibits the cellular pump that transports hydrogen ions out of the gastric mucosa. Furosemide (frusemide) inhibits electrolyte re-absorption in the ascending limb of the loop of Henle in the kidneys.

- Lactulose draws fluid into the bowel by osmosis.

- Penicillins and cephalosporins interfere with bacterial cell wall synthesis. Aminogylcosides and tetracylines inhibit bacterial protein production. Quinolones, e.g. ciprofloxacin, inhibit the enzyme that produces bacterial DNA.

(John and Stevenson, 1995; Shepherd, 2002a)

Drug metabolism

This is the breakdown of drugs into a form that is readily excreted. However, not all drugs are metabolised before excretion: some are excreted unchanged in the urine, e.g. digoxin.

Most drug metabolism is carried out in the liver by enzymes; some metabolism also takes place in the gut lining, kidneys and lungs (Goodinson, 1986b; Shepherd, 2002b).

Why is drug metabolism important?

- Most drug interactions occur during metabolism.

- The drug metabolites can exert a pharmacological effect: some drugs are inactive until metabolism has occurred, e.g. cyclophosphamide and prednisolone.

- The body can only metabolise so much of the drug in a set period of time. If the metabolism site becomes saturated, the drug action could be prolonged, causing toxicity.

- Drug metabolism breaks down the drug into a water-soluble form ready for excretion (Goodison, 1986b).

Some drugs can induce or inhibit the production of enzymes that influence the metabolism not only of that drug but also of other drugs. If the inducing or inhibiting agent is removed, toxicity may occur.

Examples

- Carbamazepine and phenobarbitone induce liver enzyme production, which decreases the effect of warfarin, thereby increasing the risk of thrombosis.

- Phenytoin and carbamazepine enhance the metabolism of oral contraceptives, reducing their effectiveness.

- Barbiturates induce enzymes in several pathways, increasing their own metabolism and also that of drugs such as phenytoin and tricyclic antidepressants.

- Cimetidine, omeprazole and amiodarone inhibit liver enzyme production, which increases the effect of warfarin, thereby increasing the risk of bleeding.

(Goodinson, 1986b; *Nursing Times*, 1994a; John and Stevenson, 1995; Shepherd, 2002a)

Clinical relevance

- A patient who is stable on aminophylline decides to give up smoking. With nicotine no longer present, liver enzyme production reduces, drug metabolism slows and plasma levels of aminophylline increase. This may result in toxicity.

Other factors that affect drug metabolism are:

- Age – especially important in the elderly and the young.
- Alcohol consumption.
- Diseases that affect liver function – half-life of the drug will be prolonged and the effects of the drug can be prolonged or enhanced.
- Smoking – nicotine induces liver enzyme production.
- Genetic factors – genetic abnormalities in enzyme systems that control drug metabolism can affect responsiveness to drugs, e.g. malignant hyperpyrexia in response to the administration of halothane and suxamethonium (Goodinson, 1986b; John and Stevenson, 1995).

Excretion

Drug that is free in the plasma can be excreted via the kidneys (in urine) or the liver (in bile and subsequently in faeces); this is called plasma clearance. Drugs can also be excreted in saliva and sweat and via the lungs (anaesthetic gases) and in breast milk (Goodinson, 1986b; John and Stevenson, 1995).

> **Clinical relevance**
>
> ❖ Excretion of some drugs may discolour urine and faeces. This can cause distress in patients if they are not warned to expect this, particularly if the discoloration is red as people often mistake this for blood.

What is plasma half-life?

This is the time taken for the plasma concentration of a drug to reduce by 50%. Drugs with a shorter half-life will therefore need to be given more often.

> **Clinical relevance**
>
> ❖ Drugs cleared via the kidneys are cleared in proportion to creatinine clearance, and may therefore accumulate in a patient with renal failure. Examples include aminoglycosides and vancomycin.
> ❖ Haemodialysis readily removes water-soluble drugs.
> ❖ Peritoneal dialysis readily removes lipid-soluble drugs.
>
> (Goodinson, 1986b)

- **Why do we need to measure the plasma levels of certain drugs?**

Some drugs (e.g. gentamicin, theophylline, digoxin) have a very narrow range of plasma concentration within which they are effective and safe. If the plasma concentration is too high, toxicity can occur; if it is too low the treatment will fail. Plasma levels of many drugs are also influenced by other factors, e.g. hypothyroidism, hypokalaemia and hypercalcaemia (Shepherd, 2002a).

Adverse reactions

An adverse reaction is any response that is unintended and of no benefit to the patient. There are two types of adverse reaction (Shepherd, 2002a):

- **Type A/augmented reactions**: These are related to the normal action of the drug, and are often caused by affinity to more than one type of receptor, e.g. the effects of amitriptyline as described earlier.
- **Type B/bizarre reactions:** These are reactions unrelated to the drug's normal action or dose, and are unpredictable, e.g. anaphylaxis.

Some groups of people are at greater risk of adverse drug reactions (Kelly, 2001):

- **Pregnant women**
  Many drugs cross the placenta and may cause congenital abnormalities or affect the growth and functional development of the fetus, e.g. steroids, narcotics and anaesthetics. Drugs such as aspirin given shortly before or during labour can affect labour or the baby after delivery. Consult the relevant appendix in the *British National Formulary (BNF)* for up-to-date information.

- **Women who are breastfeeding**
  Most drugs will be present in breast milk in small amounts and therefore have potential effects on the baby. However, only a few drugs are contraindicated. These include cyclophosphamide, cyclosporin, bromocriptine and lithium. Consult the relevant appendix in the BNF for up-to-date information.

- **Neonates, infants and children**
  Drug distribution, action, metabolism and excretion in this group may differ from that in adults, because of differences in size, proportions, constituents of the body and physiology, hence adverse effects are more likely.

- **Older people**
  Drug distribution, action, metabolism and excretion in this group are influenced by the normal physiological changes that occur with age and result in deterioration in homeostatic mechanisms and organ function and changes in body composition. Coupled with this, there may be multiple pathology that necessitates the taking of multiple drugs, and reduced functional ability, which may affect the administration of drugs.

Kelly (2001) provides a more detailed rationale of adverse drug reactions in these groups. It is well worth a read to increase your understanding of the specific effects.

What are the principles of safe practice for giving medication?

In 1986 the UKCC produced an advisory paper on the administration of medicines, which stated that first-level nurses and midwives should be considered competent to administer medicines on their own, and be responsible for their actions in so doing. Involvement of a second person would need to occur only if a learner was being taught, the patient's condition made it necessary, or in some exceptional circumstances.

Healthcare institutions vary in their policies regarding the checking procedures for drugs, and the number of people who should be involved. Children's services often require two people to check drugs before administration, because of the often complex calculations required. Many institutions require two people to check intravenous (IV) and cytotoxic drugs because of the rapid effect of the drug, and the implications should an error occur.

Action	Rationale
Before administration, read prescription chart carefully. Ensure that you know what the drug is for, the usual dose, side-effects, contraindications and any special instructions or precautions.	To check that the prescription is written clearly (in indelible ink) and accurately. It is part of the nurse's role to act as the last line of defence against errors. The doctor may have overlooked potential interactions and may have made a mistake in the dose or route (*Nursing Times*, 1994b, NMC, 2002d).
If prescription chart is unclear in any way, return to prescriber for clarification.	To reduce the risk of error (Dimond, 2004; *Nursing Times*, 1994b).
Check that patients' details are clearly written on the chart. If there are patients with the same or similar name, a warning label should be attached to the chart.	To provide sufficient information to check that medicines are given to the correct patient.
If more than 1 chart, ensure that charts are clearly marked 1 of 2, or 2 of 2, as appropriate – merge all onto one chart at earliest opportunity.	Ensures that everyone is aware of the existence of more than one chart to reduce the risk of missed doses.
Check that the allergy status of the patient is indicated. If the patient has no allergies, this should be clearly stated as 'no known allergies' (NMC, 2002d).	To ensure that patients are not prescribed drugs to which they have an allergy.
Check that the patient's weight is clearly written if any medicine is prescribed where the dose is related to weight.	
Check each prescribed medication for: • Name of drug • Route of administration • Dose • Start date • Signature of doctor • Any special instructions (e.g. with food) • Time of last administration • Time due for administration (NMC, 2002d).	To ensure that the correct drug is given by the correct route in the right dose at the right time. Some drugs, e.g. antibiotics, are only given for a short course; as the nurse administering the drugs you should request a review of the need for a drug if it has been given for longer than the recommended period. To check that dose has not already been given.

continued opposite

Figure 5.1. Drug administration flow chart.

The NMC (2004c) *Guidelines for the Administration of Medicines* is a guide for practitioners in the principles of safe practice and should be used in conjunction with local policies and procedures.

Nurses should incorporate the five 'rights' of drug administration (*Nursing Times*, 1994b) into their practice:

- Use the *right* drug
- Give to the *right* patient
- Give the *right* dose
- Give by the *right* route
- Give at the *right* time.

Figure 5.1 provides a step-by-step guide to the stages that should be followed in the checking and administration of medicines.

Action	Rationale
Check for any coexisting therapy, particularly in the 'as required' section.	To ensure the same drug or constituent of a drug has not been prescribed in more than one section – risk of overdose (NMC, 2002d).
Check drug against prescription: • Name of drug • Dose of tablet/capsule/syrup etc • Calculation (if any) • Expiry date (NMC, 2002d).	To ensure that correct dose and drug is given.
Check patient's identity against prescription chart and name bracelet. Always ask the patient to state their name, address and date of birth; do not ask 'Are you Mr ....', as a confused, hard-of-hearing, or anxious patient may answer yes to this question when it is not his/her identity.	To ensure that correct patient receives the correct drug (*Nursing Times*, 1994b; NMC, 2002d).
Obtain patient's consent and administer the drug.	Patient's consent is required for all treatments (NMC, 2002d).
Record that the drug has been administered. Where supervising a student in the administration of medicines, you should clearly countersign the signature of the student (NMC, 2002d).	To indicate that the drug has been given and to prevent the dose being given again.
Record if the drug has not been given for any reason and inform the prescriber.	It may be necessary to alter the route of administration or review the need for the drug (NMC, 2002d).
Instruction by telephone to administer a previously unprescribed substance is not acceptable (NMC, 2002d).	Risk of unclear instructions or misunderstanding. If absolutely necessary, repeat instructions back to prescriber and ensure that you have a second witness; both of you should record the instructions.

Figure 5.1 (cont'd). Drug administration flow chart.

Staff Nurse Survival Guide

Some common problems in the administration of medicines

- **Conflict with prescriber:** What would you do if you felt that the dose of a drug that was prescribed for a patient was unusually high, and when you questioned the doctor who had prescribed it he confirmed that this was the dose he wanted? You are personally accountable for your actions: if you are still concerned, you should check with a more senior doctor and seek advice from your pharmacist. Other sources of information that are available to you include the BNF and any local prescribing guidelines (Dimond, 2004).

- **Illegible writing:** You cannot read clearly the name of the drug that has been prescribed, but it has been administered by several of your colleagues at previous administration times. If you are in any doubt, do not administer the drug, and check with the prescriber, senior doctor or pharmacist first. If you do not check an illegible prescription and an error occurs, you will be equally liable (Dimond, 2004). After checking with the prescriber, always request that the prescription is rewritten. Many institutions clearly state in their drug policies that prescriptions must be written in capital letters in indelible ink.

- **PRN (as required) medication:** These are drugs prescribed by a doctor, but administered to the patient at the nurse's discretion, based on their assessment of the patient. They typically include analgesics, sleeping tablets, indigestion medicines, etc. Often, insufficient information is provided when these drugs are prescribed, such as the maximum amount that can be given in 24 hours and intervals at which they can be given (Dimond, 2004). You must be aware of the limitations of these drugs. You should check not only the time of the last dose, but also the total that has been given in the last 24 hours, e.g. a patient prescribed paracetamol 1 gram, which can be given every 4–6 hours, with a maximum of 4 grams in 24 hours. If the patient requests pain relief at 06.00 h, 10.00 h, 14.00 h and 18.00 h, the 24-hour limit will have been reached. If the patient requests further doses at 4-hourly intervals, he/she will have received an overdose of the drug. When administering drugs prescribed on the PRN part of the prescription chart, you should always check the regularly prescribed drugs to be certain that there are no contraindications. An example of this would be the prescribing of PRN paracetamol and a regular prescription for co-codamol, which could result in an overdose of paracetamol being administered.

- **Instructions by word of mouth:** The NMC (2004c) makes it clear that 'instructions by telephone to a nurse to administer, even in an emergency situation, a hitherto unprescribed drug cannot be supported.' One of the main difficulties in taking instructions over the phone is proving what was said. If it is essential to take a prescription over the phone, the nurse receiving the instruction should repeat back to the doctor what has been said and also have a witness present; this should be recorded immediately in writing. However, this should always be a last resort (Dimond, 2004).

* **A dose is missed:** If a dose is missed, for whatever reason, this should be recorded and reported as soon as possible. The implications for a missed dose are:

  - recurrence of symptoms
  - lower plasma levels of the drug
  - diminished effect of the drug.

This is especially important for drugs such as insulin, anticoagulants, and drugs for epilepsy, myasthenia gravis and Parkinson's disease (*Nursing Times*, 1994b). Some of the most common reasons for missing a dose are:

- nil by mouth
- nausea/vomiting
- patient states that they do not require the drug.

Some drugs can still be administered when the patient is nil by mouth before surgery or a procedure; advice should be sought about which drugs can be given, or they should be administered when the patient returns from the procedure. If the patient is unable to take anything orally for a longer period of time, the need for an alternative route of administration should be discussed with the prescriber.

If patients state that they do not require the drug, an assessment should be made as to whether the drug should be changed to a PRN prescription or whether the patient requires educating about the need to take the drug regularly for maximum benefit. A common example is a patient who stops taking lactulose as soon as they have had their bowels open, and then restart it when they have not had their bowels open for 3–4 days. These patients will require educating about the need to take lactulose regularly and be shown how the daily dose can be titrated until a regular pattern of bowel action is achieved.

Hazardous drugs

Drugs are not without risk to the person administering the drugs and you need to be aware of specific hazards and how you can minimise the risk to yourself.

Drugs can present a hazard to the person preparing or administering them through dermal contact, inhalation or inadvertent ingestion (Worthington, 2002).

Hazardous drugs, as defined by Worthington (2002), are drugs that:

- cause cancer
- damage the developing fetus (teratogenic) or impair fertility
- cause chromosomal breakage
- produce serious organ toxicity at low doses.

The main groups of hazardous drugs (Worthington, 2002) are:

- cytotoxic drugs
- antiviral agents
- sex steroid hormones
- immunosuppressive drugs
- anaesthetic gases.

The above list indicates those drugs which are particularly hazardous; however, repeated exposure to any drug can present a hazard to the nurse. It is therefore vital that you adhere to safe handling practices, not only to protect yourself from harm, but also to prevent you becoming sensitive or resistant to the drugs.

Safe handling practices

- Hazardous drugs should be prepared as much as possible in a properly functioning biological safety cabinet by properly trained staff.
- Always wear protective clothing – gloves when handling any drugs, and aprons, goggles and masks as required.
- Dispose of hazardous drugs in leak-free containers.
- Ensure that you receive proper training in dealing with spillage.
- If using aerosolised hazardous drugs, ensure adequate ventilation and respiratory protection for healthcare workers (Worthington, 2002).
- Never handle tablets because of the risk of sensitisation (*Nursing Times*, 1994b).
- Never eat or drink in drug preparation areas.
- Always wear protective clothing when handling body waste, as some hazardous drugs can be still be present in body fluids several weeks after administration.

What do I need to know about drug calculations?

The calculations that nurses are required to do in relation to drug administration can be complicated, and often cause anxiety.

You should be able to make calculations without the use of a calculator, since reliance on a calculator can result in errors. You should always calculate a rough estimate before using a calculator.

> '*Complex calculations may require a second practitioner to check to minimise the risk of error. Use of calculators should not act as a substitute for arithmetical knowledge and skill.*'
> (NMC, 2004c)

When two people are involved in the calculations, each should make the calculation separately and agree on the result to minimise the risk of error.

The following are a few simple formulae to assist you in the more common calculations, followed by a series of questions for you to test yourself (the answers are provided at the end of this section).

Manually controlled infusions

You do not have a pump to administer an infusion of 1 litre of 0.9% sodium chloride over 6 hours, and need to be able to set the correct rate of drops per minute.

$$\text{Rate} = \frac{\text{volume (in drops)}}{\text{time (in minutes)}}$$

To be able to calculate the rate, you need to know how many drops per millilitre the administration set delivers. This information can usually be found on the packet, but a rule of thumb would be:

Clear fluids = 20 drops/ml
Blood = 15 drops/ml

To calculate the volume in drops, you need to multiply the volume (in ml) to be administered by the number of drops per ml; to calculate the time in minutes, you need to multiply the time over which the fluid has to be administered by 60, the number of minutes in an hour. The formula therefore becomes:

$$\text{Rate} = \frac{\text{volume (in ml)}}{\text{time (in hours)}} \times \frac{\text{no. of drops per ml}}{60 \text{ (no of minutes in an hour)}}$$

So, if we take the above example of 1 litre of saline over 6 hours:

$$\text{Rate} = \frac{1000 \times 20}{6 \times 60} = \frac{20000}{360} = \frac{500}{9} = 55.55$$

You would therefore round up the result to 56 drops per minute.

Mechanically controlled infusions

You have a volumetric pump to administer an infusion of 1 litre of 0.9% sodium chloride over 6 hours, and need to be able to set the correct rate of ml per hour.

Rate = volume (in ml) ÷ time (in hours)

So, taking the above example of 1 litre of saline over 6 hours:

Rate = 1000 ÷ 6 = 166.66…

You would therefore round up the result to 167 ml per hour.

Sometimes, especially when administering antibiotics, we have to administer smaller amount over periods such as half an hour, 20 minutes or 100 minutes.

If we have 100 ml to administer over 30 minutes, this is relatively simple, since we know that 30 minutes = 0.5 hour:

Rate = 100 ÷ 0.5 = 200 ml per hour

But what if we have 250 ml to administer over 100 minutes?

$$\text{Rate} = \frac{\text{volume to be administered (in ml)}}{\text{time (in minutes)}} \times 60 \text{ (minutes in an hour)}$$

$$= \frac{250}{100} \times 60 = 150 \text{ ml per hour}$$

Drug dose calculations

We often have to administer IV drugs where the dose is different from the amount in the ampoule, and we need to calculate the amount we need to draw up.

For example, we need to administer 320 mg of gentamicin, which is manufactured in ampoules of 80 mg in 2 ml. The formula for this type of calculation is:

$$\text{Amount (in ml)} = \frac{\text{what you want}}{\text{what you've got}} \times \text{what it's in}$$

What you want   = 320 mg
What you've got = 80 mg
What it's in   = 2 ml

Therefore the calculation is: (320 ÷ 80) x 2 = 8 ml

Test yourself on the following calculations

Try them without using a calculator first: the answers can be found at the end of this section (pages 99–100).

Some basic calculations

1. Multiply:

(a) 83 x 10   (b) 83 x 100   (c) 83 x 1000

2. Multiply:

(a) 0.0258 x 10   (b) 0.0258 x 100   (c) 0.0258 x 1000

3. Divide:

(a) 3.78 ÷ 10   (b) 3.78 ÷ 100   (c) 3.78 ÷ 1000

4. Divide (write answers in decimals):

(a) $\dfrac{569}{10}$ (b) $\dfrac{569}{100}$ (c) $\dfrac{569}{1000}$

5. Complete the following:

(a) 1 gram = ... milligrams
(b) 1 milligram = ... micrograms
(c) 1 litre = ... millilitres

6a. Change 0.78 grams to milligrams
6b. Change 34 milligrams to grams

7a. Change 0.086 milligrams to micrograms
7b. Change 294 micrograms to milligrams

8a. Change 2.4 litres to millilitres
8b. Change 965 millilitres to litres

Drug doses for injection

1. An injection of morphine 8 mg is required. Ampoules on hand contain 10 mg in 1 ml. What volume should be drawn up for injection?

2. Digoxin ampoules on hand contain 500 micrograms in 2 ml. What volume is needed to give 350 micrograms?

3. A patient is ordered 16 mmol of potassium chloride. Stock solution contains potassium chloride 25 mmol in 10 ml. What volume is needed?

4. A patient is to be given erythromycin 120 mg by injection. Stock vials contain 300 mg/10 ml. Calculate the required volume.

5. Stock heparin has a strength of 5000 units/ml. What volume must be drawn up to give 6500 units?

6. Pethidine 85 mg is to be given intramuscularly as premedication. Stock ampoules contain pethidine 100 mg in 2 ml. Calculate the volume required.

7. A patient is to receive an injection of gentamicin 350 mg. IV ampoules on hand contain 80 mg/2ml. Calculate the volume required.

8. A patient is prescribed bumetanide 0.8 mg intramuscularly. Stock ampoules contain 2 mg/4 ml. What volume should be drawn up for injection?

9. Folinic acid 365 mg is ordered. Stock on hand contains 400 mg in 8 ml. What volume is required?

10. Stock calciparine contains 25 000 units in 1 ml. Calciparine 15 000 units are ordered. What volume is required?

Doses of tablets

1. A patient is ordered co-trimoxazole 960 mg orally. Stock on hand is 480 mg tablets. Calculate the number of tablets required.

2. How many 30 mg tablets of codeine are needed for a dose of 0.06 grams?

3. A patient is ordered ranitidine 225 mg orally. In the ward are 150 mg tablets. How many tablets should be given?

4. Ordered: codeine 15 mg orally. Stock on hand: codeine tablets 30 mg. How many tablets should the patient take?

5. Penicillin 625 mg is required. On hand are tablets of strength 250 mg. How many tablets should be given?

6. A patient is prescribed 75 mg soluble aspirin. On hand are 300 mg tablets. How many 75 mg tablets should be given?

7. Ordered: 0.25 mg digoxin orally. Digoxin is available in tablets containing 125 micrograms. How many such tablets should the patient be given?

8. Captopril 25 mg is prescribed. How many 50 mg tablets should be given?

Doses of syrups/suspensions

In each of the following examples you are given the prescribed dose and the strength of stock mixture on hand. Calculate the volume to be given.

1. Ordered: ampicillin 500 mg
   On hand: syrup 125 mg/5 ml

2. Ordered: chloral hydrate 1500 mg
   On hand: mixture 1 gram/10 ml

3. Ordered: chloramphenicol 750 mg
   On hand: suspension 125 mg/5 ml

4. Ordered: trimethoprim 200 mg
   On hand: mixture 50 mg/5 ml

5. Ordered: erythromycin 1250 mg
   On hand: suspension 250 mg/5 ml

6. Ordered: aspirin 900 mg
   On hand: mixture 150 mg/5 ml

7. Ordered: penicillin 1000 mg
   On hand: mixture 250 mg/5 ml

8. Ordered: chlorpromazine 35 mg
   On hand: syrup 25 mg/5 ml

9. Ordered: penicillin 1200 mg
   On hand: mixture 250 mg/5 ml

10. Ordered: erythromycin 800 mg
    On hand: mixture 125 mg/5 ml

Infusion rates

1. A patient is to have 800 ml Hartmann's solution over 10 hours. The IV set delivers 15 drops/ml. Calculate the rate in drops/min.

2. 325 ml of blood is to be given over 4 hours. The IV set delivers 15 drops/ml. Calculate the rate in drops/min.

3. 800 ml of fluid is to drip at 50 drops/min. How long will the fluid last if the IV set delivers 15 drops/ml?

4. Half a litre of fluid is being given at 25 drops/min. The IV set delivers 15 drops/ml. What time will it take to give this amount?

Answers to drug calculations		
Basic calculations		
(1a) 830	(1b) 8300	(1c) 83000
(2a) 0.258	(2b) 2.58	(2c) 25.8
(3a) 0.378	(3b) 0.0378	(3c) 0.00378
(4a) 56.9	(4b) 5.69	(4c) 0.569
(5a) 1000	(5b) 1000	(5c) 1000
(6a) 780 mg	(6b) 0.034 g	
(7a) 86 µg	(7b) 0.294 mg	
(8a) 2400 ml	(8b) 0.965 litres	

> **Answers to drug calculations (cont'd)**
>
> *Drug doses for injection*
> (1) 0.8 ml; (2) 1.4 ml; (3) 6.4 ml; (4) 4 ml; (5) 1.3 ml; (6) 1.7 ml; (7) 8.75 ml; (8) 1.6 ml; (9) 7.3 ml; (10) 0.6 ml
>
> *Doses of tablets*
> (1) 2; (2) 2; (3) 1.5; (4) 0.5; (5) 2.5; (6) 0.25; (7) 2; (8) 0.5
>
> *Doses of syrups/suspensions*
> (1) 20 ml; (2) 15 ml; (3) 30 ml; (4) 20 ml; (5) 25 ml; (6) 30 ml; (7) 20 ml; (8) 7 ml; (9) 24 ml; (10) 32 ml
>
> *Infusion rates*
> (1) 20 drops/min; (2) 20 drops/min; (3) 4 hours; (4) 5 hours

What are the routes of drug administration?

The manner in which drugs are administered determines whether the patient benefits from the treatment or suffers adverse effects.

> **Examples**
>
> ❖ Furosemide (frusemide) given too quickly intravenously can cause deafness.
> ❖ Oral penicillin given with food is not well absorbed.
> ❖ Over-application of topical steroids causes thinning of the skin, which increases absorption and leads to systemic side-effects.
>
> (Shepherd, 2002b)

Two factors determine whether the drug will reach its intended site of action in the body:

- bioavailability of the drug
- how the drug is administered.

Bioavailability

This is the proportion of the drug that enters the systemic circulation and reaches the site of action. If administered by the IV route, 100% bioavailability is achieved. Although some drugs administered orally (e.g. ciprofloxacin) are well absorbed and achieve a bioavailability similar to that achieved by the IV route, most drugs given orally do not and require an oral dose significantly higher than their IV dose. One of the reasons for this is that first-pass metabolism occurs with oral drug administration. Drugs are absorbed across the intestinal mucosa and enter the portal circulation; they then pass through the liver, where a proportion of the drug is metabolised, reducing the bioavailability of the drug.

Some enzymatic breakdown also occurs in the intestinal mucosa and lungs (Goodinson, 1986a; *Nursing Times,* 1994b; John and Stevenson, 1995; Shepherd, 2002b). Some drugs, e.g. gentamicin, do not easily cross the gastrointestinal tract mucosa and oral absorption does not occur (John and Stevenson, 1995).

Example

❖ The beta-blocker propranolol is given in a dose of 40 mg or above orally, but in a dose of only 1 mg intravenously.

Oral drug administration

This is the most frequently used route, the most convenient and the most economical. The solid forms of oral preparation are very stable and the dose is accurate. Absorption from the gastrointestinal tract occurs mostly in the small intestine where the surface area is greatest.

The oral route, however, is not without problems and many factors can make absorption from the gastrointestinal tract unpredictable. For example, the presence of food in the gastrointestinal tract can alter:

- pH
- gut motility – increased motility means less time available for absorption.
- emptying time of the stomach – if emptying time is delayed, the drug will not reach the intestine and the rate of absorption will therefore be reduced.
- rate and extent of drug absorption:
  - cephalexin, amoxicillin and isoniazid are less well absorbed in the presence of food
  - flucloxacillin taken on a full stomach will only achieve 30–50% absorption and should therefore be given 1 hour before food or on an empty stomach
  - tetracycline is less well absorbed in the presence of dairy products
  - other drugs, such as aspirin and prednisolone, should be given with or after food to decrease gastric irritation

(Goodinson, 1986a; John and Stevenson, 1995; *Nursing Times,* 1994b; Shepherd, 2002a, 2002b).

Malabsorption syndromes such as Crohn's or coeliac disease can either increase or decrease drug absorption. Absorption may be reduced if a patient has diarrhoea or constipation (John and Stevenson, 1995).

The patient may be unable to swallow tablets or capsules. In this situation, there are a few options available:

- Some tablets can be broken into smaller pieces or crushed. Some tablets are specifically designed to dissolve or to be chewed. Enteric-coated or sustained-release tablets should never be crushed or chewed as this damages the release-controlling mechanism, resulting in the whole dose being absorbed at once rather than over a number of hours. Toxicity or overdose may occur if the whole dose is absorbed at once, and suboptimal treatment will result if the dose is not absorbed at all (*Nursing Times*, 1994b; John and Stevenson, 1995; Shepherd, 2002b).

- Some capsules can be opened and the contents sprinkled onto food or mixed with a small amount of water.
- Many drugs are available as syrups or in dispersible form.
- Caution should be taken to ensure that patients do not leave tablets to dissolve in their mouth if they are intended to be swallowed whole, as this could cause burns to the oral mucosa.

Nursing implications

- Timing of drug administration is important to ensure optimum treatment, especially when the drug must be given before or with food.
- Always seek advice from a pharmacist regarding the crushing, chewing or opening of capsules.
- Tablets containing drugs that are gastric irritants are enteric coated so that the tablet remains intact in the stomach before passing into the small intestine, where the coating is dissolved. Patients should not take antacids that alter the gastric pH at the same time as enteric-coated tablets as the coating may dissolve in the stomach, causing irritation and ulceration of the gastric mucosa.

(John and Stevenson, 1995; Strachan, 2001; Shepherd, 2002a)

Sublingual drug administration

This is not a common route; perhaps the most well-known drug to be administered this way is glyceryl trinitrate (GTN) for angina. The tablet is placed under the tongue and allowed to dissolve. The drug is rapidly absorbed into the systemic circulation and avoids first-pass metabolism in the liver (*Nursing Times*, 1994b; John and Stevenson, 1995; Shepherd, 2002b).

Rectal drug administration

This route also avoids firt-pass metabolism in the liver. The benefits include:

- Valuable means of localised drug delivery to the large bowel, e.g. rectal steroids for the treatment of ulcerative colitis or Crohn's disease.
- Delivery of antiemetics in a patient who is unable to take oral drugs because of nausea and/or vomiting.
- Delivery of drugs in a patient who is unable to swallow.
- Delivery of drugs that could be inactivated by gastric secretions.

(Goodinson, 1986a; *Nursing Times*, 1994b; Shepherd, 2002b).

Nursing implications

- ❖ Some people find the rectal route unacceptable – you should check its acceptability with the patient.
- ❖ The presence of hard faeces in the rectum will affect the absorption of a drug by this route; drugs should be placed against the mucosa and not in the centre of faeces.
- ❖ Rectal administration should be avoided in patients:
  - with a low platelet count – risk of bleeding
  - with neutropenia – risk of mobilising bacteria
  - who have recently undergone rectal and/or anal surgery.
- ❖ Caution should be taken in patients with large haemorrhoids.
- ❖ Correct storage of rectal drugs is important as suppositories may melt at high temperatures.

(John and Stevenson, 1995; *Nursing Times*, 1994b; Shepherd, 2002b)

Topical drug administration

This is the direct application of drugs to the tissues to treat localised disease. Advantages include:

- drug availability at the intended site of action
- reduced systemic side-effects.

Examples of topical drug administration include:

- ointments/creams to the skin
- eye drops
- nose drops
- ear drops
- inhaled bronchodilators
- vaginal pessaries.

Topical administration can also be used to deliver drugs to the systemic circulation, usually over a sustained period of time – in some cases several weeks. This is achieved via transdermal patches. Drugs administered by this route include GTN, fentanyl and hormones (*Nursing Times,* 1994b; John and Stevenson, 1995; Shepherd, 2002b).

Nursing implication

- ❖ Always wear gloves when applying topical preparations to reduce the risk of absorption through your skin.

(John and Stevenson, 1995)

Staff Nurse Survival Guide

Parenteral drug administration

This includes subcutaneous (SC), intramuscular (IM) and IV drug administration. All of these routes avoid first-pass metabolism in the liver (Goodinson, 1986a).

Subcutaneous and intramuscular drug administration

These routes allow a 'depot' of a drug to be inserted into the muscle or adipose tissue, from which the drug is released into the systemic circulation over time and achieves a slow, sustained action. Some oil-based injections given this way need only be administered monthly or even 3-monthly (Shepherd, 2002b).

> **Nursing implications**
>
> ❖ The patient must be assessed for suitability for these routes, as the state of the patient, e.g. presence of shock or oedema, can sometimes lead to unpredictable absorption.
>
> ❖ The nurse must be aware of the underlying structures, such as nerves, which can be accidentally hit if the drug is not injected in the correct place. Knowledge of the correct technique and placement is paramount. Avoid SC or IM injections in patients with:
>   - liver disease
>   - clotting abnormalities
>   - low platelet counts.
>
> (John and Stevenson, 1995)

Sites for SC injections:

- outer aspect of the upper arm
- mid-abdominal wall
- outer aspect of the thigh

(Gilsenan, 2000).

SC injections are traditionally given at a 45°angle, but with the new shorter needles, such as those used for insulin injection, a 90° angle should be used.

The skin should be pinched to lift the adipose tissue away from the muscle, as inadvertent injection into the muscle will result in more rapid absorption of the drug. It is not necessary to aspirate the needle after insertion into SC tissue; in fact, aspiration before the administration of heparin increases the risk of haematoma (Workman, 1999).

Sites for IM injection:

- deltoid muscle of the upper arm
- gluteus maximus muscle

- gluteus medius muscle
- anterior quadriceps muscle

(Workman, 1999; Gilsenan, 2000).

It is important to inject the drug into a well-perfused muscle to ensure rapid systemic action. Patient assessment will influence the choice of site and should include:

- patient's general status – muscle mass
- age of the patient
- amount of drug to be given.

Sites should be rotated if repeated injections are required.

The needle should be inserted at a 90° angle and aspirated for 5–10 seconds to check that a blood vessel has not been accessed; discard if blood is obtained. Inject slowly approximately 1ml every 10 seconds to allow the muscle fibres to expand and absorb the drug. Wait 10 seconds before withdrawing the needle, to allow the drug to diffuse into the muscle. Do not massage the site as this encourages the drug to leak out (Beyea and Nicoll, 1996; Workman, 1999).

Complications of IM injections include:

- pain
- muscle atrophy
- fibrosis
- nerve damage
- tissue necrosis
- gangrene

(Workman, 1999).

Nursing implication

❖ Regular swabbing of the skin with alcohol before subcutaneous or intramuscular injections can result in hardening of the skin. If the patient is physically clean and the nurse has maintained a high standard of hand hygiene and asepsis throughout, there is no need to clean the skin. However, if you do clean the skin, you should allow 30 seconds for it to dry as injection of alcohol causes a stinging sensation.

(Workman, 1999)

Intravenous drug administration

This route should only be used if no alternative route is available, since it is the most inconvenient route for both the patient and the practitioner. It also carries the greatest risk of all the routes of administration, owing to:

- the immediate onset of action
- often complex calculations
- often complex dilutions
- the need for extra care with administration rates, e.g. furosemide (frusemide) should not exceed 4 mg/min to prevent transient hearing loss; vancomycin should not exceed 10 mg/min to reduce the risk of hypotension, shock and cardiac arrest
- possible incompatibilities with other IV solutions
- use of infusion devices
- risk of infection – aseptic technique required
- harm to patient from extravasation

(John and Stevenson, 1995; Shepherd 2002b).

Protein preparations should not be shaken, but should be rotated gently to prevent denaturation and frothing (*Nursing Times*, 1994b).

> **Nursing implications**
>
> ❖ Most NHS trusts require practitioners to undergo additional training before being allowed to administer IV drugs.
>
> ❖ You should ensure that before administering any IV drug, you are knowledgeable in the action of the drug, side-effects, and whether dilution is required before administration. Some drugs can cause severe phlebitis if not diluted adequately before administration.
>
> ❖ You should also be aware of the guidance provided by the Nursing & Midwifery Council (2002d) and ensure that, if you are administering the drug, you have either prepared the drug or witnessed the preparation:
>
> > *'It is unacceptable to prepare substances for injection in advance of their immediate use or to administer medication drawn into a syringe or container by another practitioner when not in their presence.'*
>
> Exceptions to this include an already established infusion, and medications prepared in pharmacy and labelled for an individual patient.

What are the ethical issues in drug administration?

When patients refuse their drugs, the nurse faces a dilemma: should she disguise the medicines in food or drink or just not give the medication, which might result in deterioration of the patient's health? Is covert administration ethical or legal? This method of administration has been common practice over the years in many settings where the nurse is acting alone.

The UKCC (2001) produced a position paper on the covert administration of drugs in an attempt to assist practitioners in decision-making; however, some feel that this area still presents an ethical and legal minefield and that more work is required by the NMC to clarify the position of nurses (Carlisle, 2002).

There are ethical, legal and pharmaceutical issues that need to be considered in the covert administration of drugs. Ethically, is it right to trick a patient into taking medication? There may be circumstances when, by doing so, you save a life or avoid substantial harm. If you did administer a medication covertly, can you be prosecuted under criminal law or the Human Rights Act? (Treloar *et al*, 2000, 2001) The UKCC (2001) advises that disguising medicines in the absence of informed consent may be regarded as deception. A clear distinction should always be made between those who have the capacity to refuse medication and whose refusal should be respected, even if the decision adversely affects their health, and those who lack this capacity. The pharmaceutical properties of a drug may be changed if the preparation is crushed and added to food or drink.

Nursing implications

❖ You should never feel that you have to make a decision alone to administer drugs covertly, and it is recommended that you follow these steps if the patient does not have the capacity to make an informed decision:

- Discuss with the multiprofessional team
- Discuss with the patient's relatives
- Respect any previous instruction left by the patient
- Consult local policies or, if not available, ask to see them
- Seek advice from your employer's legal advisors
- Maintain good records of decisions and actions taken
- Agree a method of administration with the pharmacist
- Remember that the capacity to consent can fluctuate and should be regularly reassessed
- Remember that you are accountable for your actions.

(UKCC, 2001)

How can I avoid drug errors?

'It is worth bearing in mind that administering drugs in a busy ward can be rather like driving, in that it is easy to allow a sense of routine to take over and not concentrate fully on the job in hand. Like driving, mistakes can happen at any time, and they may prove fatal.'

(*Nursing Times*, 1994b).

Lack of knowledge is a common cause of error (Cavell, 2000); however, care also needs to be taken when two patients have the same or a similar name.

There are two main types of error (*Nursing Times*, 1994b):

Error of omission:
Where the nurse unintentionally fails to give a prescribed drug.

Error of commission:
Where the nurse administers a drug that was not prescribed, or an excessive dose of a prescribed drug.

In the past, drug errors were often linked with blame and led to disciplinary action. This led to fear of reporting errors and the potential harm to patients going unchecked (Department of Health, 2000a). Today the NHS promotes an 'open no blame' culture to encourage reporting. All incidents, however, do require a thorough investigation to be able to distinguish between errors that were concealed or occurred as a result of reckless or incompetent practice, and those that occurred as a result of pressure of work and where there was immediate, honest disclosure in the patient's interest (NMC, 2004c).

The government document *An Organisation with a Memory* (Department of Health, 2000a) identified common errors that have resulted in litigation claims. They include:

- incorrect or inappropriate drugs
- wrong drug
- administration error
- failure to warn the patient of the side-effects.

The new National Patient Safety Agency (NPSA) has been charged with the task of ensuring that reporting of errors, and lessons learnt from them, are disseminated throughout the NHS (Shepherd, 2002c).

Risk management strategies use 'near misses' as a way of reducing systemic errors, such as ensuring that sufficient information is available to prescribers, promoting electronic prescribing to reduce the risk of errors from poor handwriting, and integrating pharmacists into clinical teams to anticipate errors rather than discover them (Cavell and Hughes, 1997; Audit Commission, 2001).

Nursing implications

You can avoid making drug errors by following some simple principles:
- Always check the prescription carefully against the drug to be administered.
- Always check the patient's identity against the prescription chart, even if it is your own mother or a patient you have known for many years.
- Be assertive to prevent interruptions during the drug administration process; ask them to wait until you have finished.
- Always follow local policies and procedures; they are there to protect the patient from harm and yourself from errors.
- If you do make an error, report it immediately to minimise harm to the patient.

What are the alternative and new initiatives in drug administration?

Self-administration

Receiving medication from the nurse by the traditional drug round method while in hospital encourages dependent behaviour in patients, and rarely includes education of patients about their drugs (Leadbeater, 1991). If patients are not fully informed about their medications they are unlikely to comply fully. This could result in:

- slower recovery from illness
- increased risk of secondary health problems
- poorer quality of life
- deterioration in the patient's condition
- re-admission to hospital
- premature death

(Shepherd, 2002c; Williams, 1991).

The reasons why patients fail to comply include:

- forgetting to take the occasional tablet
- taking too high a dose
- failing to get the prescription dispensed, because of apathy, lack of understanding of why the medications have been prescribed, or inability to pay for the prescription
- they feel better and therefore stop taking the drug before the end of a course
- undesirable side-effects
- complexity of the regimen – multiple drugs
- a behaviour change is required while taking the drugs, such as no alcohol and dietary restrictions.

(Williams, 1991; Shepherd, 2002c)

Compliance can be improved by:

- counselling and education
- assessment of the patient's ability to administer the drugs
- provision of aids to facilitate administration, e.g. easy-to-open bottles, measuring cups and spoons, dosette boxes
- providing adequate information about each drug

(Williams, 1991; Shepherd, 2002c).

Self-administration by patients or carers while in hospital is supported by the NMC (2004c) and the Audit Commission (2001), and fits in with the philosophy of self-care and patient education.

The advantages of self-administration include:

- enables patients to become responsible for their drugs in preparation for discharge, while having access to professional support
- improves patients' knowledge of their drugs
- increases compliance
- improves communication between the patient and the nurse
- enables patients to keep to their home routine and usual times, e.g. being able to take their medication with food, or at night, without having to wait for the drug round

(Leadbeater 1991, Shepherd 2002b, 2002c).

Self-medication is not just a matter of handing the drugs over to the patient or carer; it requires a change in your role in the drug administration process – from one of administering to one of assessing, supervising and educating.

Nursing implications

❖ If patients are not going to administer their own medicines on discharge from hospital, they will not be suitable for self-administration in hospital.

❖ Patients should be assessed for their suitability to administer their medicines, including manual dexterity and memory – aids could be utilised if any difficulties are identified. Discuss with your pharmacist.

❖ Patients' competence should be reviewed periodically.

❖ Use patients' own medicines wherever possible, as they will already be familiar with the packaging and names.

❖ Medication for self-administration should be labelled with the patient's name and clear instructions on how and when to take the drugs.

❖ Complete any documentation that your institution requires – this may be in the form of a consent form or disclaimer. A record should be made in the patient's care plan that he/she is self-administering.

❖ Patients should be supplied with a record card that contains all details of the medicine to be taken, including:
  - name of the drug
  - purpose
  - how the drug should be taken
  - when it should be taken
  - how long it should be taken for
  - any special precautions or storage requirements
  - side-effects.

❖ You should check, on a daily basis or more often if required, that patients are administering their medicines correctly, and keep a record of this checking procedure.

> ### Nursing implications
>
> ❖ The patient's drug chart should be clearly marked that the patient is self-administering to ensure that any change to regimen is communicated promptly to the nurse and the patient.
> ❖ If any changes are made to the prescription, the patient will require educating about the additions. If any drugs are discontinued, these should be removed from the patient's bedside immediately.
> ❖ You should ensure that patients are aware of their responsibility for the safety and secure storage of their medicines, which should be kept in a locked cupboard or drawer at their bedside.
>
> (Leadbeater, 1991; Shepherd 2002b, 2002c)

Patient group directions

Many clinic areas used to have 'standing orders' – a list of drugs that a nurse could administer to a patient without a doctor's prescription. However, the Crown report (Department of Health, 1999a) showed that these had no legal standing. This led to the publication of a new statutory instrument (Department of Health, 2000b), which introduced patient group directions (PGDs).

What are PGDs?

PGDs are 'written instructions for the supply or administration of medicines to groups of patients who may not be individually identified before presentation for treatment' (Department of Health, 2000b).

This is *not* nurse prescribing and should not be confused with it.

Why do we need PGDs?

PGDs are needed to improve services to patients: they reduce delays in treatment by ensuring that the right treatment is delivered by the right professional at the right time. Patient choice should be taken into account: if patients prefer to wait for a prescription from a doctor, that choice should be respected (Spyropoulos, 2002).

How do I know what I can administer?

The legislation is very clear about how a PGD should be produced and what it should include:

- the name of the business to which the direction applies, e.g the ward within a hospital
- the date the direction comes into force and the date it expires

- class of health professional who may supply or administer the medicine
- signature of the doctor/dentist and pharmacist who have agreed to the direction
- signature of the appropriate representative of the organisation
- description of the medicine to which the direction applies
- clinical condition or situation to which the direction applies
- description of those patients excluded from being treated under the direction
- description of the circumstances in which further advice should be sought from a doctor and arrangements made for referral
- details of appropriate dosage and maximum total dose, quantity, pharmaceutical form and strength, route and frequency of administration
- relevant warnings, including potential adverse reactions
- details of any necessary follow-up actions and the circumstances
- a statement of the records to be kept for audit purposes

(Department of Health, 2000b).

Are there any drugs that cannot be included under a PGD?

Yes – controlled drugs cannot be used with a PGD.

Can any nurse supply or administer the medicines included within a PGD?

No – only fully competent, trained professionals can operate within a PGD (Spyropoulos, 2002). Most organisations require a nurse to undertake additional training before she/he can operate within a PGD. You should check the requirements of your own trust.

Nurse prescribing

This section will provide only a brief summary of nurse prescribing since the nurse is expected to have several years of experience in the clinical specialty and be practising at a senior level before being able to undertake this role.

In 1992 the Medicinal Products: Prescribing by Nurses Etc Act was passed. This was amended in 1994 to provide a revised list of products in the Nurse Prescriber's Formulary, which applied only to community nurses.

In 1999 the Crown report (Department of Health, 1999b) recommended that prescribing authority should be extended to other first-level nurses.

In 2001 the Department of Health (2001e) produced an extended formulary that included:

- All general sales list medicines
- All pharmacy medicines
- Some POMs, to enable nurses to prescribe in four areas:
  - minor ailments
  - minor injuries
  - health promotion
  - palliative care.

In 2002, education and training for nurse prescribers commenced. It provided a comprehensive programme over a 3-month period. This included 25 taught days, accompanied by learning in practice supported and assessed by a mentor. Since nurse prescribers are accountable both legally and professionally, they have to possess greater knowledge of pharmacokinetics, pharmacodynamics, anatomy and physiology and the disease process, the patient's circumstances, medical history and current medications (Courtenay and Butler, 2002).

In 2003 the regulations were amended to include 'supplementary prescribing'. This allows nurses who undertake a course similar to the 'independent prescribing' curriculum to prescribe from the medical formulary (with the exception of controlled drugs). Before this can happen, a management plan needs to be written in conjunction with the supplementary prescriber, the medical practitioner and the patient. This new initiative will be of particular benefit for patients with chronic medical conditions.

Your status as a nurse prescriber must be recorded on the NMC register (NMC, 2004c).

What are the principles of patient medication?

Personal notes and contacts

Chapter 6

How do I look after a student?

Paul Pleasance

- What is the role of the mentor?
- What is involved in teaching a student?
- What is involved in assessing a student?

What is the role of the mentor?

Mentors, supervisors and assessors

There is probably greater emphasis on the support of students undertaking practical placements now than used to be the case (Department of Health, 2000b, 2000d; English National Board [ENB] for Nursing, Midwifery and Health Visiting, 2001a). A variety of new roles have been developed, including practice (or clinical) experience coordinators, lecturer practitioners, clinical educators, training leads and practice educators. In some areas the contribution of senior students to supporting more junior students has also been officially recognised. However, there is little doubt that the most important person in the everyday practice-based life of the nursing student is still the staff nurse. She/he is there, all the time, working as the primary nurse and fulfilling the role to which the student aspires. It is the staff nurse who is likely to be allocated the task of 'looking after' the student. So how do you do it? What skills do you need? And how can those skills be developed?

First, it may be helpful to clear up a few misconceptions and give some working definitions. Many nurses will be familiar with the concepts of supervisors and assessors; indeed, these terms are still sometimes used, although, in the eyes of the statutory body, they have been replaced by the concept of the mentor.

Generally speaking, nursing students can and will be supervised by a whole range of professionals during the course of their studies, including nurses, midwives, social workers, teachers, play therapists, operating department practitioners and doctors. All of these people, provided that they understand the nature, kind and content of the nursing curriculum, can make an important contribution to the learning experience of the student. While those professionals who are not first-level registered nurses can also contribute to the assessment of students (by providing feedback, for example), the formal assessment of achievement of nursing competence must be completed by the first-level registered nurse – functioning as the assessor. This is the person whom the Nursing & Midwifery Council (NMC) now refers to as a mentor.

It would perhaps, therefore, be useful to replicate the official definition of the mentor (ENB, 2001b):

> *'The term "mentor" is used to denote the role of the nurse, midwife or health visitor who facilitates learning and supervises and assesses students in the practice setting.'*

In case there is any doubt left in your mind, as you look back at your own nurse education programme, remember that all students are responsible for their own actions and inactions, but cannot be professionally accountable for those actions until they are registered. This means that the person who is supervising the student effectively carries that burden; you therefore need to distinguish in your mind the difference between *direct* supervision and *indirect* supervision. The latter reflects the fact that once the supervisor (and the student) are both confident in the ability of the student to carry out specific duties, the student can go and do them without having somebody looking over her/his shoulder (but the supervisor is still accountable for the student's actions). If the student and/or supervisor are not confident about the required activity, then it is essential that the student is directly supervised until both parties are happy about it.

There are other situations, e.g. the checking or administration of drugs (so long as this is permissible under local policy), when the student should only ever be allowed to work under direct supervision – in other words, even if the student becomes quite skilled at it, she/he can't do it alone until fully registered.

Preparation of mentors

Until August 2001, there was no standard, universal pattern for the preparation of supervisors and assessors of preregistration nursing students. There was a variety of courses, ranging from the ENB 998 'Teaching and Assessing in Clinical Practice' through to individual study days. Any and all of these forms of preparation probably provided an entry onto the local 'register of supervisors and assessors'. Since 1 September 2001, all of that officially ceased with the introduction of the new 'Preparation of Mentors' programme, which replaced the ENB 997/998 and, for community staff, the 'Community Practice Teacher' course. A word of reassurance, however: if you were already on the database of supervisors and assessors (perhaps through having completed ENB 998, or the Community Practice Teacher course, or other local preparation course) you almost certainly do not have to undergo any further study (i.e. the Preparation of Mentors course) in order to function as a mentor. By all means check with your local university, but, basically, if you were on the register you stay on it (subject to regular updating and continued professional registration).

Nurses who have not previously been on the register of supervisors and assessors now have to undertake the new course before they can be the official named mentor for nursing students. Obviously, you will need to check out local information about the course in your area, but the standard entry requirements are as follows (ENB, 2001b):

- Current registration with the NMC (first or second level).
- Other professional and academic qualifications and experience commensurate with the context of care delivery (you will need to find out how that is being interpreted in your area).
- Normally, at least 12 months full-time (or equivalent part-time) experience.

While widely welcomed, these changes have created some new challenges for all the stakeholders in the nursing education process. The most significant challenge is perhaps that, with the best will in the world, in many areas the new Preparation of Mentors courses simply cannot, in the short term, prepare enough new mentors to meet the demand.

This has led to the introduction of a range of innovative approaches, including the development of distance/open learning versions of the course. Furthermore, the valued contribution that continues to be made by professional nurses (and others) who are not recognised mentors has been acknowledged by the introduction of concepts such as 'team mentoring' and 'associate' or 'secondary' mentors. These are professionals who have undergone some basic preparation for the role and are able to supervise nursing students with confidence, and who contribute to the assessment process by providing feedback both to the student and to the named mentor, who should then complete the formal part of the assessment.

Arguably this chapter might be seen as underpinning the preparation that associate or secondary mentors might receive, but hopefully it will provide some back-up and revision for people who are doing, or have done, the full mentor preparation programme.

Mentoring a student

We know that the mentor is a person who facilitates learning and supervises and assesses students while they are undergoing practice experience. But what does this mean in real terms?

Lloyd Jones *et al* (2001) add 'general support' and 'acting as a role model' to the list, and also make the point that the word mentor is probably a misnomer, since the relationship between mentor and student is inevitably too short lived to be really meaningful (being limited by the duration of the placement). This type of mentor also usually lacks one of the historical characteristics of the role, namely that she/he should be selected by the student, presumably on the basis of a rapport that either potentially or actually exists.

There is perhaps a distinction between *informal* and *formal* mentoring. Undoubtedly the statutory body is talking about the latter, but it would be inappropriate not to acknowledge, in our professional practice, the importance of the former, i.e. informal mentoring. If we accept this, we might then add other dimensions to the role – such as knowledgeable friend, helper, advocate, challenger (Daloz, 1986), coach, counsellor and guide (Morton-Cooper and Palmer, 1993) and perhaps even confidante (Jarvis and Gibson, 1997).

Creating a relationship

It may be considered obvious that the quality of the relationship between the student and the mentor is vital if mentorship is to be successful. However, Jarvis and Gibson (1997) suggest that the relationship does not have to be of a certain type in order for this to take place – arguably the relationship might be as informal or formal as the types of mentoring that take place. They conclude that:

> 'Mentorship is about exercising this characteristic [openness] in genuine dialogue, so that ultimately both [the mentor and the student] develop and feel needed through the relationship'

One of the most important aspects of building the relationship and making mentorship work is regular contact (Lloyd Jones *et al*, 2001) so that the two parties can start to feel comfortable and confident about each other. The most obvious way is to try to ensure that you work together as frequently as possible, especially if the student is able to work alongside you while you are involved in giving care. This approach has three benefits:

- It allows the student to learn by observing first hand.
- It demonstrates to the student that you have sufficient confidence in your own skills and are happy to have those skills scrutinised.
- It can begin to demonstrate that you trust and respect the student as a colleague.

Opportunities to work together are made easier by the fact that it is now usual for the student to experience care across the full 24-hour, seven day a week span from very early in their course. So, with appropriate negotiation, it should be possible to go some way towards having matching duty schedules. This also helps to fulfil the statutory obligation that the mentor is required to:

> '...directly observe the student's achievement of intended learning outcomes for a period of sufficient length to allow valid judgements to be made.'
>
> (ENB, 2001a)

On the other hand, the assessment focus and the need to 'get the signature in the box' (and the implicit 'power' dynamics that this imposes) can distort the relationship and make it hard for the student to be honest, open and to admit to shortfalls in knowledge. Care is clearly needed to keep a balance between the various components of the role and to ensure that the relationship is a healthy one. It is perhaps no coincidence that the first UKCC Advisory Standard for the mentorship preparation programme is 'the development of effective relationships based upon mutual trust and respect' (ENB, 2001b).

In a report of her research into effective mentoring, Spouse (1996) suggested ways in which the relationship between the mentor and student can be optimised. These included such basic things as the mentor initiating social interactions, which, as well as promoting trust, show a sense of warmth – in other words, having a chat and demonstrating a personal interest in the student while, at the same time, being able and willing to share her/his own personal feelings and experiences and thus being seen as a real person in the student's eyes. Spouse (1996) also found that student stress was inversely proportional to the degree of student familiarity and friendliness demonstrated by the mentor. Gray and Smith (2000) summarised this neatly when they concluded that having a good mentor usually coincides with having a good placement.

Rather more anecdotally, it is worth noting that I regularly have cause to ask students about their practical experiences and specifically about what they believe constitutes a good practice placement; the answers consistently come back along the following lines:

- *'They actually knew that I existed and were expecting me.'*
- *'My mentor made me feel welcome and took an interest in me.'*
- *'They seemed to like having students and wanted to teach me.'*
- *'They were always willing to ask me questions, and help me find out the answers if I didn't know.'*
- *'They didn't mind me asking questions or feel threatened by me asking them.'*
- *'They really know their stuff on that ward.'*
- *'They didn't just leave the students to fend for themselves.'*
- *'Even when they were busy, they didn't make me feel like a nuisance.'*

Perhaps equally significant in these days of staff shortages and difficulties in filling vacancies, such discussions with students often end with:

- *'I'd love to go back there to work as a staff nurse.'*

Relationships between students and mentors can be important for all sorts of reasons.

In conclusion of this section, the suggestions arising from the research by Gray and Smith (2000) into the qualities of a good mentor (as perceived by student nurses) make a helpful checklist:

- enthusiastic
- friendly
- approachable
- patient and understanding
- good sense of humour
- good role model
- professional and organised
- caring and self-confident
- good communicator
- knowledgeable about the student's course
- has realistic expectations of (plus confidence and trust in) the student's abilities
- provides regular feedback

- involves the student in activities
- spends time with the student
- shows a genuine interest in the student
- is willing and able gradually to reduce the level of direct supervision.

No-one said that being a mentor was going to be easy!

Liaising with the university

It now seems to be more widely accepted that nursing education is a shared activity between the university and the practice environment; it is not just the case that the university's students have to spend 50% of their course in practice. Perhaps more importantly, it is no longer perceived that the university 'does the theory side' and the wards 'do the practice side'. The shared ownership for the education and training of nurses has resulted in an increase in teamwork between the two sides, which itself is leading to an enhanced understanding of each other's respective needs. This is a state of affairs that we all want to encourage.

However, it can be confusing to know exactly whom to contact at the university when there is a need to do so, but safe bets will be either the module leader or the course leader. If the relevant names and telephone numbers are not recorded on the front of the assessment document or module guide that the student should have presented to you, then ask the student and record it – before there is a need to do so. The bottom line is that it doesn't really matter whom you contact at the university if you have any concerns about a student (or even if you want to say how wonderful she/he is), but be prepared for the lecturer to refer you to the right person. Please don't let that put you off. It really is important that we continue to communicate with each other.

It is also important to remember that there is a range of people who might be able to deal with any queries you may have in connection with the student and her/his course. People such as practice experience coordinators, lecturer/practitioners and allocations officers can be useful contacts. It is also not uncommon for university departments of nursing to identify specific lecturers to link with individual directorates or units. If you are not sure who your 'link lecturer' is, again it would be worth finding out and then make use of her/him.

Giving feedback

Formal assessment of students will be examined at a later stage in this chapter. *Formative assessment* is usually defined as the provision of feedback on a student's progress, which is not used to make specific judgments about the student passing or failing. A typical example of formative assessment might be:

> 'You did that bedbath on Mr X really well, and you paid particular attention to maintaining his dignity and privacy. But when we do it tomorrow, perhaps we can focus on the importance of observing and recording the state of his skin at the same time.'

It is ironic that, generally speaking, we find it easier to give praise than to criticise, and yet students often report that they don't get any feedback except about their failings – and then often too late for them to be able to do anything about it to put things right.

Two golden rules about giving feedback might be seen to emerge from this last statement:

- Don't hesitate to provide positive feedback and praise on a student's performance, i.e. don't rely on the old maxim 'No news is good news'.

- If things are not going well, then make sure the student knows about it as early as possible.

The objective here is to ensure that the student has as much time as possible to put matters right and, hopefully, avoid failing an assessment. Incidentally, you might consider it good practice to let the module leader at the university know at the same time so that she/he can support the student (and you) as well.

Students want and need feedback on both their strengths and weaknesses. They cannot engage in effective reflection and thereby refocus their learning if they do not know how well they are doing. So long as the relationship is built on mutual trust and respect (as discussed earlier), students value constructive criticism about their knowledge, skills and attitudes. The proviso is that any such feedback should be discreet and take place away from the patient (Spouse, 1996) and other members of staff.

Having made that last point, it is only fair to point out that as the mentor of the student, you will receive feedback from other members of the team (with whom the student may have worked while you were not there). It will take skill and courage to talk to the student about issues and concerns that are 'second hand' while ensuring that the student is convinced of the professional value of other supervisors reporting their opinions to you. Consideration could be given to whether the advantages of negotiating a 'ward' policy whereby, wherever practical, only the named mentor should provide detailed feedback to the student outweigh the disadvantages. It is acknowledged that, sometimes, feedback cannot wait and has to be given immediately.

What is involved in teaching a student?

One of the aspects of the role of mentor most valued by the student is the teaching component, and this is a theme that recurs throughout the research literature concerning mentorship of student nurses (e.g. Spouse, 1996; Andrews and Chilton, 2000; Gray and Smith, 2000). Students realise that there is much more to teaching than being taken away from the ward environment, perhaps to an empty side ward or day room, and being sat down to receive a lecture from one of the ward team. That is not to say that there is not a place for this on occasions: there undoubtedly is, and students enjoy it. But it is not the most important part of teaching, even though some of the principles outlined in subsequent sections might apply equally well to formal and informal teaching opportunities.

Setting learning outcomes

In the world of education the relative merits of 'objectives' versus 'outcomes' have been debated for many years. My personal feeling is that using the term 'outcomes' is probably more helpful because it encourages you to focus on what the student should learn (i.e. student centred) rather than what the teacher should teach (teacher centred) or what the student should be able to do (behavioural objectives). But that is all semantics. What is important is that consideration should be given to identifying the learning needs of the student and the learning opportunities provided by the practice placement environment.

The first question might be 'what is the student here for?' The simplest answer would be to learn how to 'do' nursing – the practice side of it. After all (you might argue), the university is there to provide the theory part. But that would undervalue your expertise as a staff nurse/mentor. You don't just know about the practical side. You are the expert with the theoretical underpinnings. So, have the confidence to see yourself as an expert (that's not the same as suggesting that you know everything): teaching a student is about being able to share that expertise – the theory and the practice.

It is a reasonable expectation that students should be able to specify what they want and/or need to learn while allocated to your area (if not, send them away to come back the next day, having identified some of their intentions). The university will have provided some guidance to the students regarding what they might expect to get out of the experience. Conversely, it is also a reasonable expectation that you will be able to identify the general and unique learning opportunities that your practice environment can provide (if not, sit down with your colleagues and do the exercise – then include your conclusions in the induction pack that you provide for all students on their first day on the ward – you do have one, don't you?). Once you have identified the learning needs of the student, and the learning opportunities of the placement, identifying learning outcomes is a marriage between the two. Of course, you will need to take into account a range of other issues to set the context of this exercise, for example:

- How long is the student to be placed with you?
- What stage of the course is the student at?
- What patients are you looking after at the moment?
- Are you planning an individual teaching session, or a day of supervised practice, or the whole allocation?
- What assessment objectives have been set that the student will have to meet?

The main value of identifying anticipated learning outcomes is that it ensures that all the players in the game – the student, you and the other members of the caring team – know and understand the purpose of the allocation. Learning outcomes can also be used to show everybody what they can contribute to the student's learning. In summary:

⌘ Learning outcomes should reflect the match between what the student wants and/or needs to know, and what learning opportunities are presented by the practice experience.

The next stage is to give some thought to how to ensure that the student achieves the agreed learning outcomes.

The learning environment

Most of our students do want to learn. Although the way they present themselves and voice their desires may be different from what we expect, the majority are still highly vocationally oriented and want to learn all the things necessary for them to become good professional nurses. This goes a long way towards ensuring solid, intrinsic motivation to learn, as opposed to the extrinsic types of motivation borne only out of such things as obligation, compulsion and fear of failure.

The classic work of Maslow (1943) would have us believe that, before effective new learning can take place, all other more basic needs should be dealt with. Despite its age, Maslow's hierarchy of needs still provides a useful template for assessing the learning environment and reminding the teacher of the considerations necessary to create a setting that will ensure that optimal learning can occur.

As further clues, a review of the literature, coupled with a discussion with students, provides the following list of the characteristics of a positive learning environment. Any person who wants to teach in a practice setting will be challenged by this list:

- a welcoming atmosphere
- the provision of high quality, evidence-based care
- repeated opportunity to practise skills under supervision
- a willingness to ask and answer questions
- a willingness to repeat explanations – once is rarely enough
- skilled, competent and confident practitioners who act as role models
- clear and effective links with the educational institution
- recognition by staff of student learning needs
- effective team leadership and good staff relations
- time dedicated to teaching – including the use of 'quiet time'.

It is no coincidence that there is much common ground between the above list and the characteristics of good mentors and good placements discussed earlier. However, one of the most significant obstacles to professional learning reported by students is that they are sometimes not sure about what they need to know. If students don't know what they need to know, it is unlikely that they will be able to identify and utilise learning opportunities effectively. It sometimes happens, then, that those students end up repeating the same activities over and over again, and fail to move on to develop other skills and knowledge.

Learning resources

In one sense, the learning environment is, or should be, an important learning resource. Knowles (1980) summarises it as follows:

> *'The psychological climate should be one which causes adults to feel accepted, respected and supported; in which there exists a spirit of mutuality between teachers and students as joint enquirers; in which there is freedom of expression without fear of punishment or ridicule.'*

There are basically three learning resources open to the student undertaking a practice experience in your area:

- you (as the student's mentor)
- other members of the interprofessional caring team
- the environment of practice itself – specifically, the patients who are there to be cared for.

This last point might create some potential ethical dilemmas since it infers that patients are being used for professional purposes, which of course they are. The fact that students are supervised in their practice effectively eliminates many of the ethical concerns, but theoretically patients can decline to have students of any kind contribute to their care delivery.

It is the role of the mentor to plan and coordinate the student's experience to ensure the best opportunities to capitalise upon what those three learning resources can offer; and if there appear to be gaps in the range of opportunities that exist, then the mentor can often create and utilise alternatives. This might mean, for example, organising activities so that the student can:

- spend some or all of a shift in a different area
- work with specific people with specific expertise
- observe techniques or procedures
- escort a patient
- follow a patient journey
- follow up some new practice experience with some theory input
- go to the library to obtain evidence to support a practice intervention.

There is another resource that students can learn from – which nurses tend to shun in their search for professional respectability – and that is knowledge derived from the history and culture of nursing. Practitioners need not be afraid of this kind of knowledge, especially when that culture embraces the concept of evidence. These are things that students cannot gain from a classroom or a book, but they are things that the professional practice-based mentor is uniquely placed to help the student to learn.

Approaches to teaching

It is beyond the scope of this chapter to try to deliver a teacher training programme that would attempt to teach the mentor how to teach her/his student. What can be achieved is probably to provide some pointers that might form a basis for reflection, out of which the mentor may start to develop a personal philosophy of how to tackle student teaching – especially within the context of some of the earlier sections under the heading of 'Teaching a student'.

For instance, it has become popular in the past 20 years or so for educationalists to debate the relative merits of pedagogy (which traditionally was used to describe the art and science of teaching, but now tends to be reserved for the teaching of children) and androgogy, which is usually reserved to describe the art and science of teaching adults.

Knowles (1973) was one of the first to describe such a theory and concluded that adults learn best when:

- the learning is self-directed
- the learning is related to their past experience
- whatever is to be learned is relevant to their everyday life
- the learning material is of a problem-solving nature.

Despite the number of years ago that these findings were first recorded, and the subsequent arguments that the differences between adult and children learning are not as clearly polarised as they might suggest, there is undoubtedly much that can and should be learned from these points.

In an ideal world, whenever we are faced with a new student, we should undertake some kind of learning styles inventory; this would enable us to make an assessment of how we should set out to teach (or facilitate the learning of) that individual student. In reality that is probably not practical, but the only thing about which there is certainty is that the student is an adult (rather than a child). My own observation is that there might be something about nursing and nurses (and, in fairness, probably about departments of nursing in universities) that causes us to tend to feel more comfortable slightly further along the continuum towards pedagogy than might be the case of other professional student groups. So don't be afraid to go down that route if it seems appropriate. The important thing is to get to know the student, so that you both feel comfortable enough within the relationship to allow flexibility in the way that things are taught – and learned.

A final point under the heading of 'approach to teaching'. Whatever approach you decide is appropriate, the emphasis needs to be upon 'learning'. You can teach and facilitate all day, but if the student is not learning, it's a complete waste of time.

What is involved in assessing a student?

The good part about assessing students is that it acknowledges the achievements of the student and shows how she/he has progressed towards the goal of registration. The bad part is that students sometimes fail. We will look at that a little later.

- **Formative assessment**
  This was defined earlier as the provision of feedback on a student's progress, which is not used to make specific judgments about the student passing or failing.

- **Summative assessment**
  Conversely, this is the judgment that the student either passes or fails, and which is therefore used to form the basis of whether or not a student can progress on her/his course and, ultimately, qualify as a nurse.

Characteristics of assessment

Each university department of nursing is required to formulate, in collaboration with colleagues from the service, assessment tools for both the theory and practice components of the course. There is a shared commitment to ensuring that all assessments are:

- **Valid:** They do assess what they are supposed to assess.

- **Reliable:** The outcomes of assessment are consistent, irrespective of when the assessment takes place and who completes it.

- **Discriminating**: A 'good' student would pass and a 'bad' student would fail.

- **Practical**: The conduct of the assessment is reasonable in terms of what it demands of the assessor by way of resources such as time and money.

It is not uncommon now for practice-based staff to be involved in the theory-based assessment of students, but it is much more likely that you will be involved in assessing the practice competence of your students. Part of your preparation to undertake the role of mentor, or your annual updating, should include developing an understanding of the nature, kind, content and use of the assessment documents used by the university in your area. If there is any doubt in your mind about what specifically is required of you, then please contact a member of the university staff (see earlier section on 'Liaising with the university') or other relevant person for guidance – before you need it. Saying to the student 'What am I supposed to do with this?' as she/he hands you the assessment book does not inspire the kind of confidence that is required as a basis for a healthy mentor/student relationship.

What is assessed?

Whichever university you are working with, you will find certain things in common. For example, all assessment documents will monitor and record the student's ongoing achievement in:

- practical skills
- intellectual skills
- interpersonal skills, including:
  – ability to work within a team
  – ability to relate to patients and their families
- integration of theory and practice
- professionalism/professional conduct.

Pitfalls in assessment

The onus is on the mentor to try to ensure that the assessment is undertaken as fairly and objectively as possible. One of the advantages of concepts such as team mentoring is that it helps to share the load of the responsibility a little: because no single mentor will be able to work with the student all the time that she/he is on duty, the wise mentor will seek and receive feedback from other members of the team, perhaps associate or secondary mentors (see earlier), on how the student has performed in relation to the above areas of achievement. At the end of the day, however, it is the mentor who has the final say as to whether or not the student has achieved the standard of performance required.

It may therefore be worth considering briefly some of the pitfalls in assessment that the mentor will need to avoid:

- **First impressions:** Sometimes the first impression formed of an individual can distort later perceptions, e.g. if the student is late on the first day, however genuine the reason, this can cause people to make wrong assumptions about other aspects of performance.

- **Halo effect**: This is where one feature or characteristic exhibited by the student (good or bad) influences or inhibits later observations, e.g. great sporting prowess, physical characteristics.

- **Stereotyping:** This is where we subconsciously classify new experiences of persons using assumptions 'learned' in the past. Most of us have to make conscious efforts not to make generalised and inappropriate assumptions about groups of people. As an example, reflect for a minute on how the general public tends to characterise nurses?

- **Recency effect:** In this situation, our overall view of a person is coloured by our most recent interactions with them. Thus, if a nurse performs badly today, we can be tempted to overlook the fact that she/he performed perfectly adequately on every preceding day, and that there may be a reason for today's performance.

- **Interpersonal attraction:** We're not talking lust here; just that if someone appeals to you, whether physically or emotionally, or if they seem to like you, then that fact can potentially influence your objectivity and make you view other aspects of their work more favourably (of course, the opposite to attraction can be equally powerful).

- **Self-fulfilling prophecy:** Eventually, it seems, people tend to behave how others expect them to. This is commonly seen in children, but many of us have experienced it in adult life. We do well if we are expected to do well; a student turns out to be useless if that's the expectation given to you (and them) by their previous assessor.

Purposes of assessment

Nobody would argue with the mentor that assessment of students is an onerous responsibility, which is in no way reduced when consideration is given to the reasons why assessment is carried out in the first place:

- to provide the student with feedback on progress
- to motivate the student to achieve outcomes
- to indicate the effectiveness of instruction
- to indicate the effectiveness of the curriculum.

These first four reasons are usually fairly easy to cope with and are unlikely to cause too much stress. However, it would be a dereliction of duty not to mention the observation that, whenever a student fails to achieve, it is always necessary for the 'teacher' (whether university based or practice based) to investigate the cause, to ensure that the performance is not in some way a reflection of the quality of support that the student is receiving.

Notwithstanding this, it is the next two reasons for assessment which potentially cause some degree of anxiety because so much depends on it:

- to indicate to the statutory body the suitability of the student to be licensed
- to safeguard the standards of nursing care by maintaining a satisfactory level of performance in future practitioners.

These are not responsibilities that anyone could take lightly. It does, however, beg the question: what happens if the student fails?

Perhaps the first point to note is that it is a difficult decision to fail a student, and it can be uncomfortable and unpleasant. We all accept that there are times when it is the only option, but that does not make it any easier. Remember that assessment is a shared activity between you and the university (and the student).

So, an important point is:

- Don't feel on your own. Don't even just keep it among your colleagues in the placement area. Make sure you discuss your concerns with appropriate staff from the university as soon as alarm bells start to ring.

This then leads to the other golden rule of assessment, namely that *a failed assessment should not come as a surprise to anybody* – not the student, not the other members of the ward team, and not the university. As part of the ongoing mentoring process, it is essential that a failure to make satisfactory progress is highlighted as early as possible, so that you and the student can sit down together to draw up an action plan (in conjunction with a member of the module team from the university) designed to help the student to overcome her/his weaknesses and, ultimately, to achieve the objectives, i.e. to help the student to pass if humanly possible.

If and when, having tried everything in your power, you do have to fail your student, it may strike you that when your last 25 students all passed satisfactorily, you never heard a word from the university. Now you've failed someone, and people are suddenly contacting you. Please don't be alarmed or surprised by this. It does not imply any criticism of you or your decision, and it certainly should not be interpreted as pressure being brought to bear upon you to pass this student (or future students). If I were the module leader, or the course leader, the reason why I would contact you would be to ensure that I had a full and complete picture of all the circumstances to present to the Assessment Board so that I could support your recommendation with confidence and authority.

It may make you feel a little better to learn that it is unlikely to be the end of the line for the student. There will be options for retrieval, although it has to be acknowledged that even final attempts are sometimes failed.

That may seem like a very negative note upon which to conclude a consideration of the ways in which practice staff can support nursing students. Thankfully, it is very much the exception rather than the rule, and the majority of students do make the grade, so long as they are given clear guidance of what is expected of them. On a more positive note, a recent inspection visit by the NMC to De Montfort University, Leicester, concluded in their feedback that:

> *'Mentors feel empowered in their role and enthused by the opportunity which they have to make a vital contribution to the education and training of nurses. This they see as an investment in their own future.'*

This is certainly the intention of the School of Nursing and Midwifery at this University.

How do I look after a student?

Personal notes and contacts

Chapter 7

How do I work with others?

Karen Jackson

- How do I work with others and become part of the team?
- How do I deal with experienced healthcare assistants?
- What am I meant to do when on a ward round?

How do I work with others and become part of the team?

Becoming part of a team

As a newly qualified nurse, becoming part of a team can be very daunting: everyone else seems to know each other and you are keen to make a good impression. The first time you have to answer the phone and say 'staff nurse' can be frightening as the person on the other end won't necessarily know whether you have been there 5 minutes or 5 months. These feelings are normal, so what can help you to function effectively?

Remember that people expect you to be asking questions and in need of support. A small notebook arranged alphabetically can act as a memory booster and save you having to ask the same questions repeatedly.

You need to spend some time understanding how the team works. This can include finding out about:

- Systems such as team nursing or primary nursing.

- Teams of medical staff, which house officers and registrars work for which consultant, and how the on-call system works. This may save you a lot of frustrating phone calls when you need someone to review a patient.

- Therapists and other professionals, e.g. pharmacists, attached to the ward or area. You need to know how to contact them: do you need to phone or will they be visiting the ward/area regularly to pick up referrals? What paperwork needs to be competed, e.g. referral cards or pharmacy request slips?

One of the roles of your preceptor is to introduce you to colleagues and multi-disciplinary team members. Try to remember their names, although this can be tricky at first. Some people have a knack for this, and others do not; name badges and ward photo boards can help to jog your memory. It may also help if you get to know a bit about them, e.g. do they have children, what are their hobbies or interests? Having this information enables you to show an interest in colleagues; they appreciate it when you can ask about a particular event, e.g. a birthday party or their child's first day at school. It can also help you to understand why a colleague may, on occasion, not be their usual self. You also need to get to know your colleagues' strengths and weaknesses, e.g. who is good at dealing with aggressive or agitated patients, those with complex needs or individuals with particular problems such as feeding. This can help you to allocate patients when you start to coordinate the ward.

You need to develop an awareness of any cliques on the ward and try to avoid being drawn into them. You need to tread a fine line between trying to get on with everyone and alienating colleagues. Keep an open mind to begin with and choose your loyalties carefully. You need to recognise that there are some people you will get on with less than others and that work is the only thing you have in common with them. Accept this and work on being polite and courteous to get you through these shifts.

One of the most useful things you can do as a new team member is to get to know your ward receptionist. She/he is often a mine of useful information and has networks of contacts in other areas, potentially saving you frustrating phone calls to get things done.

Time management and prioritisation are hard skills to learn, and when done well, like much good nursing, are invisible. A useful starting point is a sheet of paper that highlights your allocated patients and what needs doing when, for example, there are observations to be done, infusions to be read or observed and drugs to be given. This gives you an hour-by-hour breakdown of your workload.

You then need to think about how to organise yourself. Do you have to go to the same patient three times in the space of 30 minutes to do different elements of care? It is tiring for both them and you and adds to the distance walked in a shift. Think about how you can cluster care to make your contact more effective. As part of this, you need to be mindful of the workload of others and plan your own to take this into account. For example, it is no good presenting your colleague with a drug chart for intravenous (IV) antibiotics 5 minutes before they are due, and expect them to drop everything to administer them for you. This needs to be discussed at the start of the shift so that they can incorporate it into their work and can be identified from your list.

If and when you are up to date with your work, you need to think how you are going to use your time. Try to avoid sitting at the desk making casual conversation with other staff; while this can be relaxing and useful for a short period of time, there are some other very useful things you can be doing. Offer to help out your colleagues, ensure that areas are stocked up and generally tidy: think how frustrating it is when someone else has used the last one of something and not replaced it. Is there one of your patients that would appreciate a little extra time? Even just combing their hair or tidying their bed can help to develop a very therapeutic relationship. It is easy to get a label of being lazy, and very difficult to get rid of it once you have it – so it is best to avoid getting it in the first place.

Working with others

What does leadership and being in charge mean to you? These are not necessarily the same thing. Think about people you have worked with as a student. What were the leadership skills you admired in them?

These are some of the things we think are important:

⌘ Fairness in workload allocation; this includes both the number and dependency of your patients.

⌘ Being willing to help others out without being asked.

⌘ Seeing when someone is struggling and being there to support them without taking over.

⌘ Being able to take the lead when the situation demands it, e.g. in an emergency.

Aspects to consider when you are in charge are highlighted in *Box 7.1*.

Box 7.1
What to consider when you are in charge

❖ What is the skill mix of your team for that shift?
❖ How does this match the dependency levels of your patients, and do they have particular needs that only certain team members can meet?
❖ Take regular opportunities to update yourself on the state of the ward, for example:
 • which patients are in or have come back from theatre?
 • who is being discharged?
 • are there any patients who have deteriorated or are causing concern?
❖ Take steps to deal with issues as they arise, e.g. staff sickness – think about what impact this will have on subsequent shifts.
❖ Identify who is out there to help you: is there a duty manager or a bleepholder covering a floor or unit? They can often see the bigger picture, such as workloads in other areas, and help you reframe the situation. However, it is important to demonstrate that you have tried to address the situation yourself. In some cases, you may just want to run a decision about something by them; on other occasions, you may need to utilise their experience and authority because you have exhausted your options. For example, if you cannot move anyone between shifts or find anyone who is off to do overtime, you need the duty manager to agree to arranging a bank nurse.

How do I deal with experienced healthcare assistants?

You may feel quite inadequate or threatened if you are responsible for supervising some very experienced staff, such as qualified nurses or healthcare assistants. Healthcare assistants often have considerable experience and are very familiar with the ward routine. Make sure that you treat everyone with equal respect. If you gain people's respect, they will work with you and for you. Work hard and enthusiastically and you will find that staff will follow your lead. Don't be frightened or embarrassed to ask people's opinion and advice. Healthcare assistants often spend more time with a patient than you do, so make sure you ask them how they think Mrs Smith is coping with her colostomy, anxiety, new medication or whatever, and value their feedback.

Make sure you understand how healthcare assistants fit into the team. Do they have allocated patients overseen by a trained nurse or do they help out generally such as assisting with personal hygiene? You need to agree with them about who is doing what and when on a shift. There is little point in them bathing a patient when you have just spent 30 minutes doing their wound dressing. Don't be afraid to ask them to help you out. It is easy to run yourself ragged trying to do everything for all your patients because you want to be seen as a good nurse who can cope. It may sound obvious, but how you ask makes a difference. You are not there to give orders, but you need to ensure that you can make them feel that they are contributing to the smooth running of the team.

The knowledge and experience of healthcare assistants varies considerably and you should not assume that a person is competent to undertake a certain duty simply because they have worked in that area for 2 years. You may feel uncomfortable asking an experienced healthcare assistant, who may be quite a bit older than you, if they know how to do something. However, you are the accountable practitioner and you are responsible for ensuring that the person you are asking to do something has the necessary skills and knowledge to undertake it safely. They are, in turn, responsible for recognising their limitations and not taking on aspects of care that they are not competent to perform. You need to be aware of what individuals can or cannot do, and your trust's policy in assessing competence.

What am I meant to do on a ward round?

Ward rounds vary in style and duration, and so the contribution of the nurse varies. However, a key element of the role is to represent the patients' interests, either by enabling them to make their needs known or to do so yourself where they are unwilling or unable. You need to be clear that it is their view that is being articulated, and not your perception of what you think they want or need. Position yourself so that you are with your patients and not buried three deep in a crowd of medical students. Ensure that all relevant documentation is available and up to date. You may not know the observations for all the patients on the ward, but can refer to the relevant charts.

Make sure that any equipment needed is available and working. This will make you appear efficient and you will not waste time looking for things, by which time the round has moved on and you have missed your opportunity to raise your concerns about a particular patient.

Ensure that you understand any changes to treatment plans. If your area uses a ward round book, keep this up to date or keep your own notes so that changes can be communicated to colleagues, and the nursing documentation amended accordingly. Again, you need to understand how the team works. For example, are request cards and prescriptions written as the round progresses or are they all done at the end?

Be aware of infection control issues and remind medical staff to wash their hands between patients. Ensure that items such as stethoscopes are appropriately decontaminated.

How do I work with others?

Personal notes and local contacts

Chapter 8

How do I look after myself?

- How do I manage my time?
- How do I get to grips with working unsocial hours?
- What should I expect from clinical supervision?
- What do I need to know about the research process?
- What is involved in professional development?
- How can I develop my professional practice?
- What sort of post-registration course should I do?
- What are CAT points and APAs?
- What is involved in reflective practice?
- How do I prepare for an interview?

How do I manage my time?

Claire Agnew

As nurses, we spend so much of our professional life looking after others that it is easy to forget to look after ourselves. From time management, having a social life, to looking after your career, I hope these handy hints will help you through the day and point you in the right direction to achieving a happy and healthy career.

Time management

Ask yourself these questions:

- How many times have I not taken my break to get things done?
- How often do I get off work on time?
- How often do I get home and then phone work to pass on something I have forgotten?
- How long do I spend looking for things that I have lost or mislaid?

If your answer is 'sometimes' or 'frequently', then you need to develop some time management strategies to help you get through the day and feel like you have achieved your goals at the end of it. Two important aspects of time management are: being more efficient (doing something right) and being more effective (doing the right thing).

Elements of time management include prioritising, putting things off and delegation (see *Box 8.1*).

Box 8.1.
Elements of time management

Prioritising

- Write down everything that you have to do on a list and keep it with you all day.
- To help you see what needs to be done through the shift, divide the work into three main priorities and give them a ranking: 1 = urgent and important; 2 = important but less urgent; 3 = routine and low priority.
- As soon as you have completed a task, cross it off your list – nothing is more satisfying than seeing a list of tasks getting shorter.
- Be prepared to re-prioritise throughout the day; a nurse's work is never static!
- Communicate with your team regularly throughout the shift so that you all know what is going on.
- Seek help and support from colleagues as soon as you feel that you are getting bogged down with work; never be afraid to ask.
- Only keep one list – any more and you will get confused as to where you are.

Putting things off

We put things off because:
- The task is overwhelming and we are frightened of failure.
- We have little or no information to start the task, are indecisive or are unsure of priorities.
- We cannot find things, or are too busy doing unimportant things.
- We may be stressed, ill or suffering from chronic fatigue.

Ways to move forward:
- Tackle the worst or easiest task first.
- Break up the task into small manageable chunks.
- Do the parts of the task you feel you can do, then seek advice to help you complete it.

Delegation

Reasons to delegate:
- It frees more time for the jobs only you can do.
- It allows others to learn new tasks.
- It encourages motivation to become a more useful member of the team.
- The job may be better done by someone else.

Why we do not delegate:
- We feel we can do the job better.
- We do the job quicker.
- We enjoy doing the job.
- It's a habit.
- We fear letting go as someone else may do the task better.

The best ways to delegate:
- Choose the person most suitable for the job.
- Ensure that they are capable of doing the task.
- Explain the job and ask them if they foresee any problems.
- Leave them to get on with it.
- Ask them how they got on and help them deal with any unresolved issues.

(Hindle, 1998; Martin, 2000)

How do I get to grips with working unsocial hours?

Claire Agnew

Requesting off duty

We all deserve a life outside work. How often is it said that the off-duty folder rules our lives? Working with newly qualified nurses, I am never surprised that they quite often forget to book annual leave or fill out extra duty forms – this is easily done when you are getting to grips with a new job. The average person has many things to juggle throughout the day – work, partners, family, friends and further study – yet it is still important to look after your own health and wellbeing.

Box 8.2.
Points to remember when making off-duty requests

- Be fair – your team members would like to have a life as well.
- Plan ahead – there is no point expecting to get the days off you want if you don't go to book them until the week before.
- Remember, most off duty is planned 6–8 weeks ahead.
- Do not go for 4 months without a holiday or you will be too burnt out to enjoy it. Space your annual leave evenly throughout the year.
- Follow any local guidelines set for leave requests or self-rostering, such as allowing certain numbers of staff off at any one time or booking the weekend off before annual leave.

Special duty payments

Nursing is a 24-hour, 7 day a week profession; working nights, weekends and bank holidays are all part of the job. However, most nurses get some financial reward for working these 'unsocial hours', which is claimed for by filling in the appropriate forms from your place of work. It is your responsibility to fill out any paperwork related to special duty payments, and to ensure that you get the applicable shifts signed for on the days you work. You may be asked to sign forms for other staff; if you do, it is your responsibility to be certain that they worked the hours written on the form.

Maintaining a social life while doing shift work

Work should stay at work, and home should stay at home, but how easy is it to achieve this? The important thing to remember is that it is all about maintaining a balance.

Does working 12-hour shifts, doing 3 nights, having 2 days off and then back on an early shift sound like a nightmare? Welcome to the world of nursing and 24-hour care. Shift work can be difficult to get used to and it is important that you are fit to function when on duty. Gone are the days when, as a student, you could have a late night out and be able to function on the early shift the next day; you are now an accountable practitioner and need to be able to function as one.

On the other hand, if you are getting many 9–10 day stretches and a quick turn around from days to nights, and then back to days, you need to discuss this with your preceptor, mentor, ward sister or line manager. Becoming tired and stressed through shift work could affect your patient care – it is important to recognise this. You need to do something positive about it and seek out support mechanisms.

What should I expect from clinical supervision?

Claire Agnew

Clinical supervision is a process that promotes personal and professional development within a supportive relationship. It aims to promote high clinical standards and develop professional expertise by supporting staff, promoting an ethos of openness and honesty in the practice setting, and helps to develop personal awareness of strengths and weaknesses (Fowler, 1999; Wheeler, 2001; McSherry *et al*, 2002).

Sounds wonderful, but does it happen in practice? In my experience, although there are some areas that fully support clinical supervision, it is something that is often suggested after the nurse has experienced a distressing incident, and not something that is ingrained in practice. As nurses working in a stressful profession, we need to look after ourselves: clinical supervision provides an opportunity to discuss clinical issues and professional practice in a secure environment with someone whom you feel comfortable with and work towards solutions.

As you are a qualified nurse, your managers have a duty to provide clinical supervision if you request it (Fowler, 1999). Don't be afraid to ask for clinical supervision – it is not a sign of weakness. Most examples of clinical supervision are based on local arrangements that are dependent of the needs of the staff. It would not be unrealistic to expect a one-to-one meeting of about an hour once a month with your clinical supervisor. Between meetings you would be expected to reflect upon your practice and bring to the meeting any concerns that you have.

What do I need to know about the research process?

Karen Jackson

The need for evidence-based practice underpins modern healthcare provision. There has probably never been so much research taking place, so why does it seem that nursing continues ritualistic practice, with learning the ward routine crucial to your survival as a new staff nurse? How can you ensure that your practice is evidence based without alienating your colleagues?

Policies and guidelines provide a fertile area for evidence-based practice and it should be possible to identify the rationale on which any recommendations have been made. Find out when these were last updated. If you have an interest in a particular area, you may be able to get involved in work relating to it.

You need to be critical about ideas that you have read about before considering implementing them in your area. Has a piece of research been done well or are there serious flaws that limit its application? Snowball (1999) identifies five key questions to be asked when looking at research:

- what type of question is being asked?
- what sort of information would provide evidence to answer this type of question?
- what type of study would provide such information?
- what types of information resources would give access to these studies?
- hsow do we get the best out of resources?

Most research texts include guidelines on how to critique research. The main areas you need to consider are:

- **Comprehension:** Is the topic under investigation clearly identified? Is there a research question and theoretical framework? Are hypotheses to be tested stated, where applicable?

- **Compassion and analysis:** How has the literature review been done? Is the selection of methodology and methods appropriate, with evidence of the decision-making process, including issues of rigour such as reliability and validity? How have the data been collected and analysed? Have ethical issues been addressed? What limitations to the study are identified?

- **Evaluation:** Have results been interpreted appropriately, e.g. use of statistical tests or the categorisation of qualitative data? Is the interpretation of the results consistent with the findings, and can claims be justified? What implications for practice are identified?

If you want to undertake research in your area, you will need to think this through very carefully. Factors to consider are:

- whose cooperation will you need to carry out the project and change practice?
- what ethical considerations are there?
- will you receive support in terms of time and administrative support to undertake the work?

Badly done research will do nothing to enhance your reputation. It may be appropriate at this stage in your career to identify the opportunities that exist within your directorate or trust for promoting research. Many trusts have a research and development directorate, which may be able to offer advice and support. Think about setting up an interest group with like-minded colleagues to share ideas and good practice. For example, children's nurses have access to a network of local groups known as Research in Child Health (RiCH) via the Royal College of Nursing (RCN).

Consider how you can utilise opportunities such as ward meetings to introduce new ideas and consider how they might be implemented. However, you need to remember that not everyone will be so keen. It may well have been tried before and not worked; who can you persuade to give it another go or do you need to consider something else?

What is involved in professional development?

Claire Agnew

As nurses, we are accountable for maintaining a high standard of professional practice. Healthcare provision is an environment of constant change and it is vital that all nurses are able to keep up with this. Lifelong learning is a concept that gets bandied around in official-sounding documents, but within nursing it is grounded in our professional development: once you start learning, you can't stop (Nursing & Midwifery council [NMC], 2002).

Post-registration education and practice (PREP) is a set of NMC standards and guidelines that enable you to demonstrate that you are keeping up to date with developments in professional practice and embrace the concepts of lifelong learning. They include keeping a personal professional profile (see *Box 8.3*) and completing a certain amount of hours on continuing professional development.

Box 8.3
What a personal professional profile will do for you

- Help you to assess your current standards of practice
- Develop your analytical skills
- Review and evaluate past experience
- Demonstrate experiential learning
- Assist with job or course applications

The PREP Handbook is a comprehensive guide to meeting the standards set. The latest revision was published by the NMC in 2004, and is available free of charge through the NMC website (www.nmc-uk.org). I recommend obtaining this for detailed information on PREP, but here are some things to remember:

- PREP does not have to cost you any money.

- There is no such thing as an approved PREP continuing professional development activity.

- You do not need to collect points or certificates.

- There is no approved format for the personal professional profile.

- PREP must be relevant to the work you are doing or plan to do.

- It must help you provide the highest possible standards of care for your patients.

Many employers are now recognising the importance of staff development, and that by investing in this they are developing a competent, motivated and committed workforce. One way of achieving this is through appraisal or individual performance reviews (Wheeler, 2001). This provides you with the chance to sit down with your manager and plan your career; it does not matter if your career aspirations are just surviving your night shift – the important thing is that you get the opportunity to discuss your strengths and weaknesses and develop an action plan for achieving your goals. In my experience, new nurses tend to focus on the acquisition of clinical skills, getting their intravenous (IV) and cannulation certificate, and life support skills. However, it is important not to overlook your development in areas such as assertiveness, team working and time management skills.

Planning your professional development should include:

- A review of your competence.
- Setting your learning objectives.
- Developing an action plan.
- Implementing an action plan.
- Evaluation of what happened.
- Record of your study time and learning outcomes.

A framework for developing a personal professional development plan is shown in *Figure 8.2* (p.144). You can also undertake a SWOT analysis to help identify your **S**trengths, **W**eaknesses, **O**pportunities and **T**hreats. *Figure 8.1* shows an example of this.

Strengths Professional manner Easy to get on with Friendly, but assertive Clinical skills	**Weaknesses** Can't say no Leave things till the last minute
Opportunities Secondment Shadowing other staff Being a mentor	**Threats** Shortage of staff Keeping motivated Over-committing myself

Figure 8.1. Example of a SWOT analysis.

Figure 8.2. Personal development plan.

Name:	Signature:		Date:	
Job title:	Manager:		Review date:	
Career aspiration/development pathway:				
Personal learning objective	Action agreed		Timescale	Complete?

How can I develop my professional practice?

John Fowler

There are many opportunities for professional development. However, those available to you at any one time will vary depending upon:

- your vision for your career pathway
- your strengths and weaknesses
- the amount of additional time you are willing and able to invest in your development
- the culture of the area in which you work.

Some opportunities will be given to you; others may be available, but you will have to take an active part in seeking and taking them; others you will have to seek out and seize.

The development of professional practice cannot happen as an isolated event. It is part of a process of clinical experience, deepening of underpinning knowledge and exploration and development of your interpersonal skills.

Potential opportunities are listed below. Some will be available to you now, and others may become available to you over the next few years.

- **Clinical experience:** Make sure you build up an in-depth knowledge of the specialty in which you work. This includes the practice and skills of that area, and the underpinning physiological, psychological and pharmacological knowledge of the specialty and any legal and professional issues that are relevant.

- **Clinical experience:** Consider working in a different clinical specialty and broadening your clinical experience. Some clinical managers will safeguard your E grade if you change specialties by providing you with a fast-track in-service development programme for a new specialty. Be prepared to ask and negotiate these sort of conditions when planning your development.

- **Clinical experience:** Consider working in a different hospital, a different part of the country or working abroad. Obviously this option is not available to everyone and will depend upon your personal and social circumstances.

- **Clinical experience:** Length of experience is not the same as breadth and depth of experience. If you are spending 5 or 10 years in one clinical area, make sure that you become the most knowledgeable and skilled person in that specialty. Beware of becoming someone who has one year's experience 10 times.

- **Preceptorship and clinical supervision:** One of the most effective ways of making sure that you learn and develop from your clinical experience is to obtain help and advice from someone more experienced than yourself.

Clinical supervision helps you to focus on specific events and examine them in a reflective and developmental way. It is your right to have clinical supervision; this is often difficult to organise on busy clinical areas, but if you persevere it will happen and will be useful.

- **Study days and in-service training:** These are study days or short courses concerned with helping you to work in your specialty. They may involve certain mandatory courses, such as moving and handling or food hygiene, or they may be more specific to your clinical area, such as IV medication and child protection procedures. Take the opportunity not only to attend these days but also to help in their administration or, if appropriate, to lead them.

- **Short courses and open learning programmes:** There are a number of useful learning packs produced by a variety of people or institutions. For example, there may be a locally produced learning pack on 'Hip replacements' or 'Interpreting ECGs', or a more professional pack on 'Using spreadsheets' or 'Health education', or one of the *Nursing Times* or *Nursing Standard* professional development series. These courses are not usually assessed by a college or university, but are very useful in helping you to develop specific skills and knowledge that are relevant to your needs and clinical area.

- **Validated programmes:** These are usually Diplomas of Higher Education or Bachelors degrees or Masters degrees. They will involve several years of part-time study, so make sure you pick the right course for you (see the next chapter).

- **Secondment:** Occasionally, opportunities arise for a member of staff to be seconded to undertake a specific role away from her/his normal working environment. This may be within your own trust, such as transferring to another ward to cover maternity leave or to help set up a new unit. Other opportunities may include secondment to another organisation to help develop, audit or teach. These are very useful opportunities as they expose you to different ways of working and different structures for a limited period of time while maintaining the security of your employment in your original base area.

- **Research:** This may be a rather frightening option for a number of staff. However, there are many different levels in which you can be involved in research. At the simplest stage it is just becoming aware of any research that is being undertaken in your area or trust. Once you have found out what is happening, try to get involved, initially perhaps by helping out with tasks such as collecting data, sorting or photocopying. Just being involved in the research process with experienced researchers will increase your knowledge and help you to make useful contacts.

What sort of post-registration course should I do?

Nigel Goodrich and John Fowler

As discussed in the previous section, there are a number of important study days that a newly qualified nurse should undertake. These are usually organised locally, either by the unit training officer or more centrally by your employing trust or hospital. Some of these are mandatory; others are specific to the clinical area in which you are working. These study days involve particular skills or procedures that enable you to work effectively in your area. They may be concerned with IV therapy, administering medications, moving and handling, infection control etc. These are important and are usually undertaken in the first year after qualifying. As part of your preceptorship you should have identified your 'learning needs' and discussed them with a more senior member of staff. This should continue with an annual review of your performance and any training that you require – your individual performance review (IPR).

The next significant development that you should be contemplating is the mentorship course. You may already have been assisting with the support and teaching of students; however, before you can take full responsibility for overseeing a student on a placement you will need to undertake a NMC accredited mentorship course. Your local university nearly always runs mentorship courses and your application and place on the course is usually coordinated by your line manager in conjunction with a trust training officer. Most managers would expect all E grades to have undertaken, or be in the process of completing, the mentorship course, and be taking an active part in mentoring students.

Following a mentorship course, there are no specific 'rules' as to what, if any, further courses you should undertake. It is important that you seek advice before investing considerable amounts of time, energy and possibly money into further study. Some clinical areas have traditionally provided and expected staff to undergo further studies in order for them to work effectively, e.g. intensive care units, accident and emergency units, and orthopaedics, whereas other areas, such as medicine and surgery, have tended to expect staff to develop their skills and knowledge based on experience. It is important for you to find out what is currently valued in the area in which you wish to specialise. This can be part of your IPR or clinical supervision sessions.

An increasingly common national standard is the NMC's Specialist Practitioner Award. This is a post-registration award validated by the NMC, which is usually based on degree studies in an area or specialty. The Specialist Practitioner Programme prepares staff to exercise high levels of judgment and clinical decision making and is based on four key areas (United Kingdom Central Council for Nursing, Midwifery and Health Visiting [UKCC], 1994):

- specialist clinical practice
- care and programme management
- clinical practice leadership
- clinical practice development.

The majority of universities that provided undergraduate nurse training will also have a post-registration degree that is part of the NMC Specialist Practitioner Award. Most universities will have a course that enables nurses who have undertaken a pre-registration diploma of nursing to continue with degree studies and complete a degree that incorporates a NMC Specialist Practitioner Award. Building on your Diploma in Nursing, this can usually be completed part time in 2 years and will normally incorporate a subspecialty such as critical care nursing, mental health nursing or surgical nursing.

Nurses who have undertaken a pre-registration degree in nursing should also aim to complete a NMC Specialist Practitioner Award. Some universities may offer this as part of a Master's programme, but others may only offer it at first-degree level.

Once a nurse has:

- gained appropriate experience, usually a minimum of 3 years
- completed the mentorship course and is experienced in mentoring students
- normally completed a degree that incorporates a specialist area of nursing practice

then she/he could start applying for F grade or equivalent posts.

Nurses who wish to continue with their career may contemplate such posts as nurse specialist, practice development nurse or nurse lecturers, but would normally need 2 further years of experience that includes leadership and management experience and have commenced or completed an appropriate Master's degree.

It is quite probable that future nurse consultants will not only have national reputations of clinical excellence and research, but also be engaged in or have completed doctorate degree studies.

If all this seems a bit daunting and remote from patient care, don't despair. The majority of post-registration nursing courses are designed to enhance and develop client/patient care. Not all nurses need to be undertaking post-registration degrees; however, if you want to take a key role in developing client/patient care, then you need to consider how you will acquire the appropriate underpinning skills, knowledge and attitudes required to develop professional practice.

What are CAT points and APAs?

John Fowler

The majority of university degrees are structured into modules of study that are given a certain amount of points or credits. A degree is made up of a fixed quota of credits within certain subject areas. The majority of universities have agreed a set formula that allows a certain amount of transferability between different universities. Some combination of the following terminology is usually used:

Year one	certificate level	level 1
Year two	diploma level	level 2
Year three	degree level	level 3

Each year or level is made up of 120 credits. A full honours degree is made up of 120 credits at level 1 plus 120 credits at level 2 plus 120 credits at level 3, giving a total of 360 credits. Universities allocate different amounts of credits to modules of study, but the total amount will still add up to 120 for each level. Thus some universities may structure their courses as 10 modules of 12 credits each, another may have eight modules of 15 credits each and others may use a combination of 15-, 30- and 60-credit modules within their courses. The important fact is that each year or level totals 120 credits.

Courses that are run on a part-time basis have the same structure of level 1, level 2 and level 3, but level 1 may take place over 2 years rather than one year as in the traditional full-time structure.

Pre-registration diploma courses contain the academic content of level 1 and level 2 studies, but are taught over a 3-year period. This is due to the fact that nurses will not only qualify with a diploma in higher education in nursing, but also with a registered nurse professional qualification.

A number of nurses will undertake a short course or module at a university, which, although not a full degree, will normally attract credits, e.g. 30 level 2 credits or 30 level 3 credits. These are very useful and not only demonstrate continuing professional development but also the ability to study at level 3. However, simply collecting 360 credits will not necessarily be all that is required to complete a degree. A diploma or degree is made up of specific subjects, not simply the accumulation of the required number of points. Thus a degree in nursing is normally made up of modules on: research, leadership, teaching, nursing practice, physiology, psychology, sociology – all applied to health care. Simply collecting 360 credits that are only concerned with one, two or three of these subjects will not demonstrate that you have covered the syllabus of a nursing degree.

There are some specific terms associated with credits and how they can be used in a flexible way sometimes in different universities:

- **Degree**: Only a university can award a degree (360 credits).

- **Diploma of Higher Education**: Only a university can award a Diploma of Higher Education (DipHE – 240 credits).

- **Diploma**: Anyone can issue a diploma, provided that it does not say Diploma of Higher Education. So beware of paying a lot of money for a diploma that you may see advertised. The diploma may also refer to learning points or professional points – beware, these are not higher education points as awarded by a university. This is not to say that these diplomas are not worth anything; often they may provided useful information and sometimes they are validated by a professional body, but they will not count towards your degree.

- **Certificate of Higher Education**: This is awarded by a University (CertHE – 120 credits).

- **Certificate:** Anyone can issue a certificate. The same principles apply as for the diploma (see above).

- **APEL (accreditation of prior experiential learning):** This acknowledges that traditional classroom-based learning is not the only way of gaining knowledge normally associated with textbooks and classroom teaching. Experiential learning is that which we learn from experience – not simply doing the same thing again and again, but while undertaking something in clinical practice. This could involve searching the literature, writing procedures or publishing findings. If such experiential learning can be matched to a specific module of study at a university, then the student may be able to provide the evidence that they have achieved the module outcomes by an alternative route.

- **APL (accreditation of prior learning):** This is similar to APEL, but is focused on another educational institution being the source of learning. Thus someone may have undertaken a module of study on research methods while on a health studies degree. When undertaking a post-registration specialist nursing degree, the person may put in a claim that they have already met the outcomes of the specialist nursing research methods module.

- **APA (accreditation of prior achievement):** This is a general term that is usually used to cover both APEL and APL, as most claims involve both APEL and APL.

- **CAT (credit accumulation and transfer) points:** This covers the same ideas as in APEL, APL and APA, but it specifically means the transfer of a module of learning from one course or university to the course you are undertaking. Each course and university has individual regulations as to how, if at all, they allow this. Most courses will allow 20–25% of level 2 credits to be transferred in from other universities. However, at level 3 this is reduced to 15%, if it is allowed at all.

- **Advanced standing:** The normal structure for a degree is to start at year one on level 1 and work through to the end of year three. Advanced standing is the acceptance of students onto year two or year three of the degree, based upon previous APEL and/or APA. The most common example of this for nurses can be found in post-registration degrees. Most pre-registration education gives the nurse a Diploma in Higher Education (Nursing) with their professional registration. Most universities that run pre-registration nursing courses at diploma level will also have a post-registration degree that allows advanced standing from pre-registration Diplomas in Higher Education (Nursing). Thus nurses may undertake pre-registration education in one part of the country and then move to another part of the country. In their new location, they enrol on a degree course that allows them to transfer in their Diploma in Higher Education (Nursing) (240 credits) via advanced standing and then complete the equivalent of the third year of the degree.

CAT and APL are complicated yet extremely valuable structures, which many nurses can utilise. If you feel that you have credits or experience that could form part of your further studies, then seek out someone at your local university who understands the course regulations regarding APA. This may take a bit of detective work on your part, but it will be well worth the effort.

What is involved in reflective practice?

Claire Agnew

Learning is not achieved solely by having an experience or attending a study day. Learning is a result of thought and consideration – reflection about what the experience actually meant to you. The ability to reflect effectively is fundamental to the development of nursing (Andrews, 1996)

Reflection is also an important part of reviewing your strengths and weaknesses and identifying areas that need developing. It means thinking about an event, analysing what occurred, what your thoughts and feelings were about the event, and identifying what you did well and what you could learn from it. Reflection can take place in a variety of ways: a reflective journal, portfolio development, structured sessions, or the use of a framework (Hulatt, 1995).

Situations that you should reflect upon include:

- something you enjoyed or went well
- something you found difficult to deal with
- a situation where things went wrong
- a crisis or emergency
- something you do every day
- something you rarely do

(Jarvis, 1992; Haddock and Bassett, 1997; Johns, 2000).

How to reflect

How you choose to reflect upon your practice and experiences is a personal decision, although it is recommended that you choose a model that will guide you through the stages of reflective learning. Sharing your reflections with someone you feel comfortable with may provide another way of looking at the situation. Gibbs reflective cycle (Gibbs, 1988; *Figure 8.3*) provides a simple approach to reflection. *Figure 8.4* shows a framework that you may find useful.

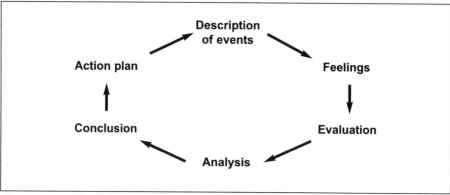

Figure 8.3. Gibb's reflective cycle (Gibbs, 1988).

Description (what happened?)
Feelings (what were you thinking and feeling?) and evaluation (what was good and bad about the experience?)
Analysis (what sense can you make of the situation?)
Conclusion (what else could you have done?)
Action plan and learning outcome
Signature ....

Figure 8.4. Framework for reflection using the reflective cycle.

How do I prepare for an interview?

Claire Agnew

Creating the right impression at interview takes preparation. For some jobs that you apply for, you may be the only applicant. Other jobs may have 10 or 20 applicants for one position. No job will be yours automatically. You need to find ways of getting the edge over other applicants, and that means preparation and presentation.

Getting an interview is reliant on your application form; it needs to be concise and comprehensive. When I shortlist candidates for interview, I look for good clear presentation. Obvious presentation points are very important, yet often missed:

- Do not write your application form in blue ink when they ask for black.
- Ensure that your handwriting is legible
- Fill in all the sections.

And I expect to see the supporting statement box filled with personal qualities: what you have done outside work that could have a positive effect on your practice, insight into the role you are applying for, and not just 'I want to work on a cardiac ward to increase my skills in dealing with cardiac arrests'. I'm looking for someone who is going to be motivated, demonstrate commitment and fit into the team.

When you get an interview, go on an informal visit where appropriate, or if it is a promotion within your existing area, arrange to see the senior nurse, training and development team or the management team. This will give you the opportunity to find out others' expectations of the role that you are applying for

---

Box 8.4
Pointers for interviews

- Arrive in good time: this will allow you to collect your thoughts.
- Research the role you are applying for.
- Dress smartly – you are a professional.
- Read the job description thoroughly and think through what the role involves.
- Think of some possible scenarios that you may be asked; where possible, answer them with previous experiences that you have learnt from.
- Think of some questions to ask the panel.
- Take your professional profile and offer it to the panel to look at.

Box 8.5
Questions you may be asked at interview

- Why do you want this job?
- How do you deal with stress?
- What is important to you as a nurse?
- What do you understand by the term clinical supervision?
- What do you understand by the term clinical governance?
- What do you understand by (insert any current government initiative or publication)?
- What qualities do you possess that you can bring to this role?
- Who or what has most inspired you?
- Tell me about a recent article you have read that has influenced your practice.

and aid your preparation; it will also help you demonstrate your interest and commitment. The RCN and *Nursing Times* websites offer very practical advice on interview preparation and preparing your CV or application form. *Box 8.4* also offers some pointers for interviews.

Box 8.5 lists some questions you may be asked at interview.

If you are unsuccessful, try not to be too disappointed. The more sought after or senior the job, the greater will be the interest and competition. Try to learn from the experience, both in terms of your character and also from how you could improve next time. Most interviewers will give you the opportunity to receive feedback; if this is not offered to you, then ask. Try to treat it positively and make sure that you are willing to listen, learn and develop.

How do I look after myself?

Personal notes and local contacts

Chapter 9

What is my role in dealing with grief, bereavement and palliative care?

- How do I talk with patients, relatives and carers?
- How do I contact relatives/carers following a death?
- What if I'm involved in caring for a terminally ill child?
- How do I care for the patient's body after death?
- How do I manage pain in palliative care?
- What are the causes of pain in advanced cancer?
- What is the analgesic three-step ladder?
- What other ways are there of managing pain in palliative care?
- How do I manage nausea and vomiting in palliative care?
- How do I manage intestinal obstruction in palliative care?
- How do I manage constipation in palliative care?
- How do I manage dyspnoea in palliative care?
- How do I manage mouth problems in palliative care?
- How do I manage the psychological care of terminally ill patients?

How do I talk with patients, relatives and carers?

Martyn Geary

How a person responds when given news of a diagnosis or prognosis will vary enormously. It will be affected by their age, gender, religion, cultural and social background and the major life experiences through which they have lived. In addition, how the person responds when given a diagnosis may echo, to some extent, how he/she has responded to and coped with previous major life events (Buckman, 1992; Higgins, 2002). It may be, for example, that the patient or his/her carer has always dealt with any form of stress or crisis by pushing it to the back of their mind, trying, as far as possible, to ignore the problem and continue with their day-to-day life as if nothing untoward had happened. If this has been the person's major coping strategy in the past, it is not improbable that he/she may demonstrate similar coping mechanisms when confronted with the news of a life-threatening condition.

Authors and researchers such as Kubler-Ross (1970) have addressed explicitly the issue of patients' coping strategies and emotional responses when confronted with 'bad news'. Kubler-Ross emphasises that people's emotions and responses very often change over time; sometimes these emotions may appear contradictory – denial and unrealistic hope for the future one day and apparently resigned acceptance of the 'inevitable' the next – as people fluctuate between different responses. The variation and changing nature of response is seen to be a perfectly normal and natural reaction to one of the most difficult situations any one of us will ever have to confront – news of a life-threatening condition. While the positive insights of Kubler-Ross' work are still as relevant today as they were 30 years ago, there are problems relating to how the insights she offers are used in clinical practice and applied by practitioners to patient care.

Writers such as Fulton and Metress (1995) argue that there is a tendency for practitioners to interpret stage theories, such as that developed by Kubler-Ross, literally and to presume that all people will pass through similar stages of 'denial', 'bargaining', 'anger' and 'depression', to arrive at the ultimate endpoint of 'acceptance'. The danger here is that practitioners may view the coping strategy displayed by an individual as one of many that they may potentially display over the course of a disease journey. While this may be true for some people, it may not be the case for others. This assumption could lead the practitioner to challenge a perceived 'unhelpful' response in the belief that once challenged it may be replaced by one they perceive to be more positively adaptive. Some people may have other coping mechanisms upon which they can draw, but for others it may mean that the only coping mechanism they have ever used is threatened. If it is taken from them, what are they to replace it with?

To avoid this situation occurring, it is perhaps helpful to view the work of authors such as Kubler-Ross as a model or guide to the overall complexities of emotional response displayed by individuals confronted with bad news, rather than see it in prescriptive terms – 'this is how people will behave'. The key, as always, is to listen to the patient or carer and to make an individualised assessment of the coping strategies and emotional responses displayed, and to plan interventions based on that assessment.

How do I contact relatives/carers following a death?

Martyn Geary

Informing relatives that a loved one has died is an understandably stressful situation for all practitioners, whatever their level of experience. The following guidelines may be helpful.

Before the death

- Record the name and contact telephone number of a person to be contacted in the event of a patient's deterioration. Do not assume that this will be the same as the next of kin. Consider recording two names to ensure that the name of an additional contact is known should the first be unavailable.
- Record the person's full name, not simply their surname – there may be people in the same house with the same surname.
- Clarify when this person might *not* wish to be contacted. For example, do

they wish to be contacted during the night? If not, ascertain the time after which they do not wish to be contacted and if there is anyone else who should be contacted in their place.

Contacting relatives/carers over the telephone

- Collect all of the relevant documentation together.
- Find a private and quiet place (preferably an office or room separate from the rest of the ward or unit) where you can make the telephone call.
- Inform colleagues of what you are about to do so that you will not be disturbed.
- Check and double check that you are about to contact the right relative or carer about the right patient – mistakes can and do happen!
- Before you dial the number, mentally rehearse what you are going to say.
- When the phone is answered, introduce yourself and ask to speak to the person concerned.
- Clarify that you are speaking to the right person. Instead of saying 'Is that Mrs Smith', say instead something along the lines of 'Is that Mrs Pat Smith, Jack's wife?'
- The phone call itself will cause alarm so do not delay in giving the news. Try to convey the information slowly and sensitively without the use of euphemisms. For example, after having established that you are speaking to the right person, you might say: 'Mrs Smith, I'm afraid I've got some bad news. There's no easy way to say this. I'm sorry to say Mr Smith has died.'
- Be prepared for a range of possible responses.
- If the person wishes to come into the hospital, ensure that you make it clear how to gain access to the hospital, particularly at night if the usual entrances are closed.
- Ask if the person is fit to drive? Ask if you could telephone anyone on their behalf.
- If they are not intending to leave for the hospital immediately, explain that you will phone back in half an hour to check on them.
- If they choose not to come in during the night, explain what needs to be done the following day.

Preparing for relatives/carers arrival

- Ensure that all staff members are aware of the patient's death and that relatives/carers are expected.
- If at all possible, try to ensure that a member of staff is allocated to the care of relatives.
- If relatives/carers are expected to arrive during the night, arrange for hospital security or portering staff to meet them at the hospital entrance and show them to the ward.
- Ensure that the allocated staff member is waiting for them on the ward and

is there to escort them to a prepared office or quiet room. Ensure that there are sufficient chairs available and tissues at hand in the room. If there is a phone in the office, divert calls to a different extension. A busy ward office is not the ideal place.
- Ensure that the nurse allocated to their care is appraised of the circumstances surrounding the death – relatives/carers are likely to have questions about what happened and the order of events. Documenting the details of events surrounding a death can also be of value if the ward or unit operates a bereavement support programme where relatives may meet with practitioners in the months following the death. Unless recorded, events around a death can be forgotten by health professionals, especially if they were not directly involved in care delivery at the time.

Being with relatives/carers

- Be sensitive to the range of possible reactions people may display.
- Remember that there is likely to be little or nothing a practitioner can say that will ease the pain that people experience. Attempting to 'reassure' can, albeit unintentionally, be interpreted as platitudes.
- Recognise and accommodate religious and cultural diversity in the way that people express their grief.
- Take your lead from the bereaved. Even if people have arrived at the hospital, check that they still wish to view the body. If so, explain beforehand what they will see when they enter the bed area or side-room. Some people may never have seen a dead body and be apprehensive as to what to expect.
- Accompany carers/relatives to the bedside.
- Check with relatives if they wish to spend time alone. Providing chairs at the bedside gives them reassurance that they will not be rushed.
- How people wish to act when with the deceased will vary. Religious and cultural factors as well as personality and the effect of grief itself will influence what people wish to say or do.
- Offer access to religious/community leader or minister if appropriate.
- Offer the opportunity for relatives/carers to speak to a member of the medical staff to discuss events surrounding the death.
- Some people may wish to kiss, hold or lie with the deceased; others may choose not to, while some may be reticent and appreciate the nurse taking the lead in touching and 'speaking' to the person who has died.
- While providing time for relatives to be alone if they wish, check regularly whether there is anything they need. Remember to point out the location of toilets and telephone facilities and offer refreshments.
- Before they leave the ward, ensure that they are given information (reinforced with written details) as to what to do and where to go to collect the death certificate and any property of the deceased. A list of support organisations should also be given.
- Ensure that all details of the visit are entered in the nursing notes.

What if I'm unable to contact the person over the telephone?

In addition to trying the number at a later time, check to see if there is an alternative contact number. If no telephone number is recorded, check with directory enquiries. Failing that, you may have to consider contacting the patient's GP, if appropriate, to request a visit to the deceased's relatives, or contact the police service who can arrange for officers to visit the address to convey the information personally. There will be a procedure for contacting the police – check this with your senior nurse manager.

What if there's an answering machine attached to the telephone?

As soon as you realise that an answering machine is attached to the phone, replace the receiver without leaving a message. This will give you time to compose yourself and to rehearse what it is you wish to say. Obviously, in the message you leave, you will not tell the relative/carer about the death, but ask them to contact the ward as soon as possible, giving the name of the person with whom they should ask to speak.

What if the person collapses with the shock of the news?

Stay calm and continue speaking to the person. If they have collapsed, it is likely they will rally within a few seconds. If this doesn't happen and they fail to respond, check in the notes of the deceased to see whether there is an alternate contact. If not, you may have to contact the police service to ask for officers to visit the person's address to check on their welfare.

What if I'm involved in caring for a terminally ill child?

Zoe Wilkes

Family-centred care

One of the major approaches when caring for a very sick child is the promotion of family-centered care. It is not only the needs of the child but also those of the whole family that need to be addressed, including those of any siblings. There is often a multidisciplinary team involved in the care of terminally ill children, providing all aspects of medical, nursing and psychological care to the family. It is important to work as a team and to coordinate and share all the treatment and care that the child and family receive. It is recognised that supporting a family during this time can be a very stressful time for the staff involved and it is often the nurse that plays a key role in helping the family and child prepare emotionally for the child's forthcoming death (Costello and Trinder-Brook, 2000). Brykcznska (1992) recognises that the nurse has a pivotal role in providing information, continuity of care and the ability to empathise on a level of sensitivity and common human understanding.

Symptom control

In a publication written for staff working in a children's hospice, Jassal (2001) advises staff to listen to the parents' views and ideas regarding symptom control, as they have become the experts in their child's care. Through a focused listening process, the level of intervention and symptom control will nearly always be established.

The symptoms listed below could be exhibited at some time in some children and should form the basis of any holistic assessment (Jassal, 2001). The assessment should be initiated as a baseline measure, and then the child should be reassessed in an ongoing manner, depending on his/her needs.

- Anorexia
- Bladder problems
- Bleeding problems
- Constipation
- Convulsions
- Cough
- Diarrhoea
- Dyspnoea
- Gastro-oesophageal reflux
- Infections
- Mouth care
- Muscle spasms
- Nausea
- Noisy breathing
- Pain
- Psychological problems
- Skin problems
- Vomiting

The treatment of many of these symptoms can be of a non-pharmacological nature, e.g. changing a child's position, altering a feeding regimen, nursing in a quiet environment. However, there will be situations where relief may only be obtained through medication. In these instances it is very important to listen to the needs and choices of the family and to work closely with the appropriate medical staff in relaying this information. It is vital that the family are given the opportunity to make informed decisions and to work in partnership with the multidisciplinary team caring for the child.

Time and emotions

It is very important to organise the environment in which the child is cared for in a way that allows time, freedom and privacy for the child and carers to express their emotions in a way that they can be sensitively cared for. This will vary depending on whether the child is in an acute hospital, a hospice or is being cared for at home.

Providing emotional support includes making sure that all staff are supported and have the opportunity to talk through their feelings as they care for the child and family. There is no right or wrong way to behave or feel in these circumstances. It is the responsibility of professionals to acknowledge their feelings in order to practise effectively. In most cases the family will look to the nurse involved in their child's care for support and guidance, therefore it is just as important that the nurse concerned seeks their own support from a source that they too feel is safe and appropriate.

How do I care for the patient's body after death?

Martyn Geary

General points

- Ensure that the death has been verified. This can be carried out by a doctor or suitably qualified senior nurse (Cooke, 2000).
- Be sensitive to the religious or cultural beliefs and wishes of the patient and their community. If at all possible, these should have been ascertained and recorded within the patient's notes before the death.
- Establish whether relatives/carers wish to view the body before or after last offices have been performed.
- In some instances this may mean that the care of the body is undertaken by family members or community leaders, or that the nurse assists as they take the lead in the last offices.
- Be familiar with your hospital/trust policy on the removal of tubes, drains and catheters as this can vary. All should be left in place, including existing dressings, if:

    - the death is unexpected
    - death occurs within 24 hours of admission or surgery
    - death is accidental or occurred in suspicious circumstances
    - cause of death is unknown
    - patient has been brought in dead
    - death may be the result of an industrial disease.

    In all the above situations it is likely that the death will be referred to the coroner (Cooke, 2000).
- Universal infection control precautions should be adopted at all times. Make arrangements with the hospital mortuary for a cadaver bag to be available if the body is leaking body fluids or known to be infected with hepatitis B, C, human immunodeficiency virus (HIV) or other communicable infection. Minimal handling of the body is recommended in such instances to minimise the risk of contamination.
- Inform other patients of the death and provide support and reassurance as necessary.
- Be aware of the needs of colleagues, particularly those who may have been directly involved in the patient's care or those with limited experience in caring for the dying and bereaved.

Undertaking last offices

- Lay the patient's body on his/her back and straighten the limbs. Place a single pillow under the head with a rolled towel on the upper chest to support the jaw.
- Use moistened cotton wool pads and light pressure for 30 seconds to close the eyelids.

- Cover any leaking wounds with waterproof dressings. If orifices are leaking excessively, packing with gauze may be required. Drain the bladder with pressure over the lower abdomen.
- As long as it is not contraindicated by religious or cultural beliefs or by the wishes of relatives/carers, wash the body and dress it in either a shroud or personal clothing.
- Mouthcare and care of dentures should also be undertaken. If the person usually wore dentures, these should usually be reinserted in the mouth. The person's previous preferences should be respected in relation to the combing and arrangement of their hair and facial shaving.
- Follow hospital/trust policy in relation to the labelling of the body. The usual procedure is to attach identification labels to one of the patient's ankles and to one of the wrists. A notification of death card is usually attached to the patient's chest before the body is wrapped in a mortuary sheet (Mallett and Dougherty, 2000).
- When wrapping the body the nurse should ensure that all limbs are secured and that face and head are covered. The sheet should be secured with tape and placed, if necessary, within a cadaver bag.
- A second notification of death card is then secured to the mortuary sheet or cadaver bag over the patient's chest.
- If relatives/carers wish certain pieces of jewellery to be removed from the body, this should be done in the presence of another nurse and be recorded on the patient's property form. If any jewellery remains on the person's body, this should be recorded on the notification of death cards that accompany the body (Mallett and Dougherty, 2000).
- Complete the appropriate nursing notes and arrange for the transfer of the body to the mortuary. Ensure that patient property is transferred (in the absence of relatives/carers) to the appropriate administrative department.

How do I manage pain in palliative care?

Wendy Taylor

What is pain?

> *'Pain is not a simple sensation, but a complex physiological and emotional experience.'* (Regnaud, 2004)

> *'Pain is whatever the experiencing person says it is, existing whenever he says it does.'* (McCaffery, 1968)

In palliative care, the effective management of pain requires:

- Thorough assessment.
- A consideration of the patient's ideas, beliefs, concerns and expectations.

- Negotiation of the management plan with the patient at all stages.
- A multidisciplinary perspective.
- A holistic approach, incorporating physical, psychological, social and spiritual aspects.
- Use of drugs, physical and psychological treatments, complementary therapies and spiritual support.

The concept of 'total pain' encompasses social, spiritual and emotional components, as well as physical, as illustrated below:

Physical influences
- Symptoms or debility
- Pathology
- Side-effects of treatment
- Cancer/non-cancer

Social influences
- Friends who do not visit
- Financial worries
- Loss of social position
- Loss of job prestige and income
- Loss of role in family
- Isolation

Emotional
Anger:
- Delays in diagnosis
- Unavailable doctors
- Treatment failure

Fear:
- Pain
- Death
- Hospitalisation
- Loss of dignity
- Loss of choice/control
- Uncertainty about the future
- Disfigurement

Spiritual
- Why has this happened to me?
- Death seen as punishment
- Helplessness
- Loss of self worth
- Why does God allow me to suffer like this?
- Is there any meaning to life?
- Can I be forgiven for the past?

Pain assessment

This should be carefully and thoroughly carried out. The following should be ascertained:

- site of the pain and any radiation (use body diagram)
- description of the type of pain, i.e. stabbing, burning, colicky
- severity of pain (scoring system can be used)
- what makes the pain better and worse
- the effectiveness of any analgesia administered and the duration of that effect.

What are the causes of pain in advanced cancer?
Wendy Taylor

Points to remember

- Not all cancer patients experience pain.
- Not every pain is due to the cancer.
- Understanding, empathy, diversion and feeling cared for are important adjuncts to analgesia.
- Attention to detail is vital – always be asking: 'Why is this happening'?

Causes of pain in advanced cancer

1. **The cancer itself**
    - Visceral from involvement of abdominal, pelvic or intrathoracic organs
    - Soft tissue infiltration
    - Bone involvement
    - Neuropathic

2. **Treatment related, e.g.**
    - chemotherapy-related mucositis

3. **Cancer-related debility, e.g.**
    - constipation
    - muscle spasm/tension
    - pressure sore

4. **A concurrent disorder, e.g.**
    - osteoarthritis
    - migraine
    - post-stroke pain

(adapted from Twycross and Wilcock, 2001).

What is the analgesic three-step ladder?

Wendy Taylor

The 'analgesic ladder' (*Figure 9.1*) provides a guidance framework for the administration of analgesic drugs.

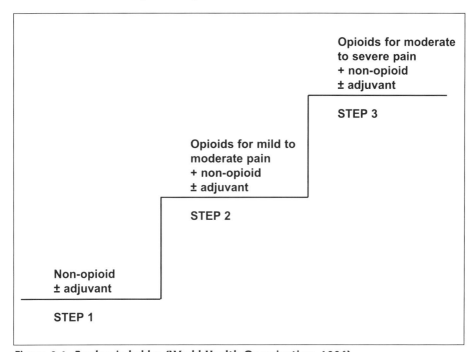

Figure 9.1. Analgesic ladder (World Health Organization, 1996).

How to use the ladder

- Start at the bottom.
- Work up in a stepwise progression.
- Use the maximum dose of a drug *before* moving up.
- Never move sideways in the same efficacy drug group.
- Titrate the drug dose upwards until the patient is pain free.
- Give analgesics by mouth whenever possible.
- Give analgesics *regularly* to prevent pain returning.
- Have realistic goals. Aim for progressive pain relief:
  - at night
  - at rest during the day
  - on movement (not always completely possible).
- Reassess constantly and adjust drugs/doses accordingly.
- Ensure that all patients have extra analgesia prescribed for transitory pain exacerbations.

(Twycross and Wilcock, 2001)

Drugs used on the analgesic ladder

NON-OPIOIDS

>   **Paracetamol**
>   **NSAIDs** (Non-steroidal anti-inflammatory drugs)

OPIOIDS

>   *Weak:*   **Codeine**
>
>   *Strong:* **Morphine** – oral strong opioid of choice
>   **Diamorphine** – parenteral strong opioid of choice

Useful alternatives to strong opioids in cases of intolerable effects with morphine are:

>   **Hydromorphone**
>   **Oxycodone**
>   **Fentanyl** – used in the form of transdermal patches

Methadone: Strong opioid (*but requires careful monitoring – usually commenced in a specialist unit*). Useful in patients with:
- adverse effects with morphine
- escalating pain despite increasing doses of morphine
- resistant neuropathic cancer pain
- renal failure.

ADJUVANTS

- Antidepressants
- Anticonvulsants
- Steroids
- Skeletal muscle relaxants
- Antispasmodics
- Bisphosphonates
- Ketamine

What other ways are there of managing pain in palliative care?
Wendy Taylor

- Radiotherapy
- Hormone therapy
- Chemotherapy
- Surgery

- Psychological, .e.g. counselling or cognitive behavioural therapy:
- Interruption of pain pathways:
  - local anaesthesia
  - nerve blocks
  - neurosurgery
  - heat pads
  - transcutaneous nerve stimulation (TENS)
- Complementary therapies:
  - acupuncture
  - relaxation
  - visualisation
  - hynotherapy
  - reflexology
  - homeopathy
  - aromatherapy
  - massage

(adapted from Twycross and Wilcock, 2001).

How do I manage nausea and vomiting in palliative care?
Wendy Taylor

There are many reasons why nausea and vomiting may occur; this can make it difficult to achieve complete control.

The mechanism of vomiting

The vomiting centre is situated in the brainstem and controls and coordinates vomiting. It responds to stimuli from:

- ***The chemoreceptor trigger zone*** – situated in the area postrema in the fourth ventricle. Stimulated by:
  - blood toxins
  - biochemical abnormalities, e.g. hypercalcaemia, uraemia
  - drugs, e.g. NSAIDs, opioids.

  Area neurotransmitters – serotonin and dopamine

- ***The vestibular nerve*** – stimulated by:
  - middle ear disease
  - motion sickness.

  Area neurotransmitters – acetylcholine and histamine

- ***The cerebral cortex*** – stimulated by:
  - anxiety
  - thoughts
  - tastes and smells

- anticipation of past remembered stimulus, e.g. chemotherapy.
  Area neurotransmitters – acetylcholine and histamine

⌘ *The vagus nerve* – stimulated by:
  - gastric stasis
  - constipation
  - gastrointestinal obstruction
  - gastric distension
  - stretched liver capsule
  - cough/excessive sputum.
  Area neurotransmitters – acetylcholine and serotonin

⌘ *Direct stimulation:*
  - Radiotherapy
  - Raised intracranial pressure

Management of nausea and vomiting

Ask: 'Why is this patient vomiting?' Identify possible causes – the treatment will depend on the cause.

Treat potentially reversible causes (Twycross, 2002), such as:

- constipation
- coughing
- raised intracranial pressure
- hypercalcaemia (if appropriate)
- gastric irritant drugs.

Use the most appropriate anti-emetic to treat the cause (see *Table 9.1*).

How should anti-emetics be administered?

The route of anti-emetic administration is important. Only use oral anti-emetics for the prevention or treatment of mild nausea. For the adequate control of nausea and vomiting, anti-emetics need to be given by:

⌘ **Suppository:** cyclizine, domperidone

⌘ **Subcutaneously:** either as a bolus injection, or using a syringe driver, with one or more anti-emetics: cyclizine, metoclopramide, levomepromazine, haloperidol, hyoscine. Once control had been achieved, oral drugs may be substituted (Kaye, 1992).

Table 9.1. Anti-emetics for use in palliative care

Drug	Affinity to neurotransmitter sites and actions
Metoclopramide	*Dopamine and serotonin antagonist* Increases gastric motility Useful for gastric stasis
Levomepromazine	*Dopamine and serotonin antagonist and antihistamine* Useful for persistent nausea and vomiting of unknown cause Sedative in higher doses
Ondansetron	*Serotonin antagonist* Useful for chemotherapy-induced nausea and vomiting Very constipating
Lorazepam and diazepam	Useful in nausea and vomiting induced by fear, anxiety, anticipation of stimuli
Haloperidol	*Dopamine antagonist* Useful in chemically induced nausea and vomiting (drugs, biochemical abnormalities, toxicity)
Cyclizine	*Antihistamine* Useful in vestibular disturbances and radiotherapy to the head and neck Very useful if you do not know the cause of the vomiting
Hyoscine	*Anticholinergic* Depresses vomiting centre Dries secretions Antispasmodic
Corticosteroids	Useful in enlarged liver and cerebral oedema, and gastric outflow obstruction
Domperidone	*Dopamine antagonist* Useful alternative to metoclopramide Acts on gut wall Does not cross blood-brain barrier, so few central effects

(Adapted from Geary, 2000)

Remember...

- *'One third of patients with nausea and vomiting need more than one anti-emetic for satisfactory control'* (Twycross, 2002).
- Use combinations of drugs, which have different actions.
- Anxiety exacerbates nausea and vomiting irrespective of the cause.
- Consider using non-drug methods:
  - distraction
  - relaxation
  - acupuncture
  - hypnotherapy.
- Give drugs subcutaneously, not intramuscularly (less painful).
- Give an anti-emetic regularly.

How do I manage intestinal obstruction in palliative care?
Wendy Taylor

Obstruction of the gastrointestinal tract can occur at any site, from the oesophagus to the large bowel. It can be partial or complete, and acute or chronic. It can be caused by a number of factors (Twycross and Wilcock, 2001):

- the cancer itself
- consequences of past treatment, e.g. adhesions
- drugs, e.g. opioids
- debility, e.g. faecal impaction
- unrelated benign conditions.

Symptoms of intestinal onstruction:

- abdominal pain (colic is common)
- vomiting
- abdominal distension
- absolute constipation (if obstruction is complete).

Management

Surgery must be considered; however, many patients are unsuitable and unfit for operation.

Nasogastric suction and intravenous (IV) fluids are usually inappropriate in prolonged inoperable obstruction.

Medical treatment

Aim: To control the symptoms and allow eating and drinking (Kaye, 1992).

- Trial of high-dose steroids may resolve the obstruction (give subcutaneously), e.g. dexamethasone.
- Nausea – use cylizine, haloperidol or levomepromazine.
- Intestinal colic:
  - stop stimulant laxatives
  - stop anti-emetics that increase gastric motility (metoclopramide, domperidone)
  - use an antispasmodic, e.g. hyoscine butylbromide
  - consider using diamorphine
  (Rudd, 2002).

A subcutaneous syringe driver can be used with a combination of drugs infused over 24 hours, e.g. diamorphine, hyoscine butylbromide, cyclizine and octreotide. Octreotide reduces intestinal secretions in bowel obstruction, thus alleviating distension and reducing the chance of vomiting and colic.

How do I manage constipation in palliative care?

Wendy Taylor

'Constipation means hard or infrequent motions' (Kaye, 1992). This is a common problem in palliative care patients – ask every patient about it.

Predisposing factors

- Poor diet and/or fluid intake
- Drugs, especially opioids, also diuretics, anticholinergics.
- Immobility
- Gut cancers
- Spinal cord compression
- Other diseases (e.g. diverticular disease)

Constipation can cause:

- Nausea and vomiting
- Impaction of faeces with overflow, causing spurious diarrhoea
- Abdominal pain
- Urinary incontinence or urinary retention (Rudd, 2002).

Treatment

⌘ If possible, reverse the cause.

⌘ Always prescribe a laxative with an opioid.

⌘ *Laxative choice:* use a softener plus a stimulant, e.g:

- senna and lactulose
- senna and docusate
- sodium picosulfate elixir (Laxoberal for resistant cases)

⌘ *Rectal intervention:*

Suppositories:
- bisacodyl (stimulant)
- glycerine (softener)

Enemas:
- arachis oil (softener)
- phosphate.

An arachis oil enema at night, followed by a phosphate enema the next morning, is useful for resistant cases.

How do I manage dyspnoea in palliative care?

Wendy Taylor

'*Dyspnoea means a distressing difficulty in breathing*' (Kaye, 1992). There is often more than one cause.

Common causes of dyspnoea in palliative care:

- Anxiety
- Lung cancer (primary or secondary):
  – obstruction of the bronchus
  – effusion
- Anaemia
- Other lung disease
- Loss of respiratory muscles
- Pulmonary embolus   (Faull and Woof, 2002)

> **Remember...**
>
> ❖ Careful assessment is required to establish the cause.
>
> ❖ Reverse the reversible (i.e. effusion, chest infection).
>
> ❖ Use drug and non-drug treatments.

Points of management

Non-drug treatments

- Explore anxieties – dyspnoea can cause panic and fear; these in turn can exacerbate the symptom. Patients often fear suffocation.
- Explain the mechanism of dyspnoea.
- Teach breathing exercises, relaxation and distraction technique.
- Adapt lifestyle; adjust to loss of role and abilities.
- Use electric fan.
- Positioning for maximal breathing.
- Listen to, support and reassure the patient.

Drug treatment

- Opioids, e.g. morphine.
- Oxygen if hypoxic and there are no contraindications.
- Nebulised saline if there is tenacious sputum.
- Bronchodilators if there is reversible airways obstruction.
- For excessive, noisy secretions – 'death rattle' – use glycopyrronium bromide or hyoscine hydrobromide. Both are powerful anticholinergics; the latter is very sedating.

How do I manage mouth problems in palliative care?

Wendy Taylor

These are common and can be distressing. Meticulous mouth care is vital in palliative care. Dentures should be removed and cleaned thoroughly daily.

Dry mouth

This is usually the result of a decrease in the amount of saliva secreted, or a change in the composition of the saliva. The most common cause is drug therapy.

Treatment Saliva substitutes:
- Oralbalance gel
- Saliva Orthana spray

Saliva stimulants:
- Chewing gum
- Pilocarpine *or*
- Bethanecol chloride (fewer side-effects than pilocarpine)

Oral thrush

Oral candidosis (thrush) can present in different forms. Features are relatively non-specific, e.g. white patches on the oral mucosa or red areas. The oesophagus can be involved, causing pain and difficulty with swallowing.

Treatment Antifungal drugs, e.g. fluconazole and nystatin. If the patient does not respond to treatment, send an oral swab to microbiology.

How do I manage the psychological care of terminally ill patients?

Wendy Taylor

To contemplate understanding how a patient who is facing death feels may seem an almost impossible task. But some emotions and fears are common experiences, and there are aspects of life that are considered important by most of us:

- work
- finance
- leisure and fun
- relationships and family
- prior experience of illness
- roles and status
- meaning of life and faith.

'It is how each patient views and copes with each of these components when facing the end of their life that drives their emotions and subsequent behaviour.'
(Faull and Woof, 2002)

Patients who are terminally ill, facing death, can experience a psychological response similar to that which occurs in bereavement. Kubler-Ross (1970) describes five stages of dying. People may experience these stages in sequence, or may oscillate backwards and forwards between the stages:

1. **Denial:** The refusal to believe the truth of what is happening.

2. **Anger:** 'Why me? Can be directed at anyone, e.g. doctor, family or a relative.

3. **Bargaining:** The patient tries to make a deal with someone, e.g. God, doctor, relative. 'If you cure me God, I promise that I'll try to be a much better person.'

4. **Depression:** The impending loss of life causes hopelessness, despair and anxiety.

5. **Acceptance:** The patient has emotionally adjusted to what is happening. The struggle and fighting is over. *Not* all patients reach this stage.

Common fears of terminally ill patients

- The process of dying
- Pain and other symptoms
- Loss of control over one's body
- Loss of control in decision making about care
- Separation from loved ones
- Rejection
- The unknown
- Dying alone
- 'Ceasing to be'
- Death itself
- Letting God down
- Unfinished business
- Dignity
- Altered body image

Remember...

❖ Sharing fears will reduce them – ask patients what they are frightened of.

How can I help patients deal with their fears?

Dying patients should always be told the 'appropriate' truth about their diagnosis; only then will they build up trusting relationships with their professional carers, and feel safe to express their fears. However, it is important for patients to retain some hope. Most patients want to talk about their diagnosis, dying and other fears.

Fostering hope

There are seven key strategies to facilitating hope (Herth, 1990):

1. The presence of a meaningful relationship
2. The ability to feel lighthearted
3. Personal attributes of determination, courage, and serenity
4. Clear aims
5. Spiritual beliefs
6. Ability to recall positive moments
7. Having one's individuality accepted and respected.

Helpful tips

What sort of relationship should I try to establish with terminally ill patients?
- Remind yourself, if possible, of what the person was like before they were ill.

How can I help patients to feel in control?
- Negotiate all proposed care with the patient, tailored to their unique individual need.
- Involve them in decision making.

Not to be alone when they die
- Patients often ask for relatives to be present, but sometimes they send them away. Some relatives are uncomfortable with being present with a dying patient and need to be given permission to leave.
- Just hold someone's hand.

Some relatives want to feel useful
- There is always something a relative can do: hold the patient's hand; clean their mouth; give drinks.

Some patients have practical issues they want to complete
- Make a will
- Have an input into their own funeral arrangements
- Restoration of an estranged relationship
- Go somewhere for one last time.
- Write letters for children to open when they are older.

Staff Nurse Survival Guide

What is my role in dealing with grief, bereavement and palliative care?

Personal notes and local contacts

Chapter 10

What else do I need to know?

❖ What are my roles and responsibilities regarding the Mental Health Act?
❖ What issues are involved in obtaining consent?
❖ What are my rights and responsibilities regarding patient records and documentation?
❖ What do I need to know about clinical governance?
❖ What are my rights and responsibilities regarding risk management?

What are my roles and responsibilities regarding the Mental Health Act?

Paul Rigby

While it is understandable to assume that roles and responsibilities relating to the Mental Health Act will concern only mental health and learning disability nurses, there are situations where nurses outside these specialties will have contact with patients subject to such legislation.

The Mental Health Act (1983) provides a legislative framework that enables people with a mental disorder to receive care and treatment. The vast majority of people accessing mental health care in inpatient settings do so on an informal basis; however, there are some who, for a variety of reasons, require legal compulsion to ensure that care and treatment are received. It is important to remember that the power to give treatment that the Act provides applies only to treatment for a mental disorder. The power to treat may be applied to a physical treatment if it is in some way related to the mental disorder, although this is not common practice and is a complex legal area.

Nurses will have contact with people who are suffering from a mental disorder such as a severe depressive illness, who will sometimes present for treatment in an accident and emergency department following an episode of self-harm. If they are willing to give their consent to treatment this is usually provided before they are referred to a specialist mental health practitioner. If this consent is withheld or withdrawn, it is important to remember that treatment can still be provided under common law provided that treatment is necessary to save life, prevent suffering or prevent deterioration in the patient's condition. This is a complex area of practice and requires good communication, effective teamwork and strong leadership.

People who are detained under the Mental Health Act will require treatment in non-mental health inpatient settings, such as a medical or surgical ward, and in such circumstances specialist nurses will provide a continuous escort. The responsibilities for the nurse in such circumstances revolve around the provision of care and treatment for the physical condition only. However, the principles of effective networking with other care providers, good teamwork, including the setting of clear boundaries in relation to roles and responsibilities and good communication, are essential if effective holistic care is to be provided.

What issues are involved in obtaining consent?

Karen Jackson

- What do we mean by consent?
- What do people need to consent to?
- Who can give consent for children, young people and adults?
- When can we proceed without consent?

We tend to think of consent as the signing of forms, but consent is generally obtained for most of what we do. Some of this is what is known as implied consent. For example, when we request to take the blood pressure of a patient, they put their arm out to enable us to apply the cuff. In this situation it is likely that the patient is familiar with what is going to happen and it is accepted that this is part of the routine. With regard to a blood test, for example, we may need to give a little more information, such as where the blood will be taken from, how much will be taken, who will take it and what it is being taken for. Here, the individual agreeing to the sample being taken would imply consent.

Consent forms are generally used for procedures that involve something more invasive, which might be done under sedation or an anaesthetic. The process involves an opportunity to weigh up the risks and benefits of having the procedure, what it involves, other options and any implications of not having the treatment. Having a signed form is a record of when discussions took place, but not proof of consent. It is not uncommon to find that your patient still has unanswered questions despite having signed the form and you will need to be proactive in ensuring that these are answered by an appropriate individual. It may be useful to help patients to identify specific questions that they have and explore the use of alternatives, such as diagrams, to enable understanding.

The issues of taking samples during surgery and the disposal of body parts were highlighted by events at Alder Hey Children's Hospital (The Redfern Report, www.rlcinquiry.org.uk/download/index.htm). The consent process therefore needs to ensure that individuals are aware of why samples are being taken. Usually this is to enable further treatment, such as samples for biopsy, but it may also be for research purposes.

With regard to who can give consent, a number of aspects need to be considered:

- **For children under 16 years of age**, consent can be given by someone with parental responsibility. Children should be involved in the consent process; this raises the concept of 'Gillick' competence, where an assessment is made of whether there is sufficient understanding and intelligence to comprehend what is proposed. The achievement of competence depends both on the child and the severity or complexity of the treatment (Dimond and Barker, 1996). Alderson (1993) notes that quite young children can give consent if they are involved in the process, particularly in the case of chronic illness, although they may still want their parents to give consent. Where the child cannot give consent it is useful to consider what elements of the process they can be involved in, e.g. having medication from an oral syringe or spoon, or what toy will accompany them to theatre. The concept of 'Gillick' competence also applies to parents under the age of 16, and they can give consent for their child if they are assessed as competent.

- **Young people of 16 and 17 years** are presumed in law to be competent, and can therefore give their own consent. It may be necessary to consider whether the family needs to be involved in the process and agreement sought on this. Young people with learning difficulties may be able to give consent if information is presented in an appropriate way, but the person with parental responsibility can give consent if needed.

- **Adults** can only give consent for themselves. In an emergency situation it is lawful to provide immediate and necessary treatment without consent. Where this is not the case, Fortes Mayer (2002) comments that it is appropriate to document the course of action being taken and why it is in that individual's best interests to proceed. In addition, a second opinion may be sought. However, cases may go to court where it is not possible for an individual to give consent. Examples include the sterilisation of young women with severe learning disabilities and withdrawing feeding in situations of persistent vegetative state. Where it becomes apparent that additional procedures are needed during a course of treatment, it is necessary to obtain further consent unless such a delay would be detrimental to an individual's life or health.

The use of interpreters in obtaining consent needs to be considered. Implications for confidentiality must be taken into account. This is particularly pertinent where the individual and interpreter both come from the same community, as they may be known to each other and the patient may be reluctant to discuss personal matters with them.

The use of family members also raises issues. Children, for example, may not understand the information given and be unable to translate it accurately. Other adults may only interpret selective information on the basis of what they think the person needs to know. Both situations mean that the individual concerned cannot make an informed decision. Remember that some things may be translated literally and the meaning lost. Some years ago, I was involved in putting together advice leaflets on HIV and AIDS. It became apparent that in one of the leaflets, anal sex had been translated as sex via the back door, not quite what was meant! At the same time, it is necessary to be sensitive to the needs of the individual and family, and in some situations the advice of senior members of the community may be sought when making a decision.

What are my rights and responsibilities regarding patient records and documentation?

Tracy Kemmitt

During your training, you would have been made aware of the many demands that have been made of you. Pressure to complete assignment work, clinical work and examinations have been juggled with having fun and everyday living. This pressure will continue for you, as it does for every qualified nurse, but it will seem more intense when you have recently qualified. You are now accountable for your actions so you will need to be more vigilant with regard to record keeping, as it is can be your way of proving that you have carried out your role as a qualified nurse.

Many nurses will argue that they do not have enough time to complete the patient records because they are giving patient care, or will say 'I don't have the time'. How often have you found the time in your average working day to visit the toilet, walk up and down or round the ward? It's all down to prioritisation of the most important events or patients. Try to complete the nursing records at the bedside, involve your patient, discuss care and answer any questions that the patient may have. Records can be written concisely and correctly in a timely manner. This combination will reduce the likelihood of complaints and increase patient satisfaction.

As a registered nurse you are signing up to being accountable for your own actions. Patient records are sought and gathered during an investigation when an incident or complaint has occurred. It is likely that your ward sister carries out this gathering in the first instance. Patient records can provide vital evidence that patients have been assessed, and care has been planned and given accordingly. In relation to wound care, for example, a well-documented assessment provides the baseline for planning and evaluating patient care. A photographic image with a grid measuring system next to it is often used in the current climate of increased complaints. The Nursing & Midwifery Council (NMC) (previously the United Kingdom Central Council for Nursing, Midwifery & Health Visiting [UKCC]) has published a range of documents which set out standards that the registered nurse has to achieve, e.g. *Code of Professional Conduct* (NMC, 2004a) and *Guidelines for Records and Record Keeping* (NMC, 2004e) (Russell, 1999).

Health care involves many different professionals, and each one has a different way of working, with different paperwork. To find out what is happening with a patient's care or progress, communication is essential, as life always seems to be in the fast lane. Verbal communication would seem the obvious way, but we only retain a limited proportion of what we hear. The longer the gap between hearing something and then trying to recall it, the greater the degree of inaccuracy. Written documentation is therefore essential. Patients' documentation can be reviewed by any healthcare professional who is charged with their care. It is also a key element whereby a third party can review nursing and medical input and also identify an inadequacy (Baestin, 1997). Accurate record keeping can provide evidence that correct nursing care was carried out

> **Points to remember**
>
> - Be sure of your personal competence.
> - Document all patient care carefully.
> - Take immediate action over patient allegations.
> - Take all complaints seriously and follow hospital policies to resolve them.
> - Check your professional indemnity insurance and make sure it is adequate and suitable for your job.
> - Check your contract of employment.
> - Follow all hospital policies and guidelines.
> - Make sure your employers know about, and authorise, all healthcare activities that you undertake.
>
> (Thomas, 2001)

at the appropriate time and may safeguard you if any complaints are made regarding patient care. As a registered nurse, it's vital that you take measures to protect yourself against liability for negligence.

The 12 steps of record keeping

1. Write it *now*, not later. We all forget details – when was the last time you went to the shops and forgot one item because you didn't write a list?

2. Record relevant points chronologically – step by step.

3. Number each page when writing extensive notes about an incident.

4. Add the patient's sticker to each page; if this is not possible, record name and hospital number – notes may accidentally fall on the floor and get mixed up or lost.

5. Always record the date, time, signature, full name in legible writing and designation after each entry. Never leave a space between your last entry and the next one – something could be added by someone else.

6. Always write clearly and legibly in black ink; blue may not photocopy.

7. Use English – obvious isn't it! Be precise, objective and clear. Imagine how it would read in court. Don't use subjective comments.

8. Made a mistake? Cross it out with one line. Use a dictionary, ask a friend! Using correction fluid over the mistake can be detected by scientific testing.

Don't let any food or drink near your patient documentation; keep it clean and presentable.

9. State the facts clearly and distinguish between fact and opinion – don't record issues that are not related to the patient or case in hand.

10. Don't blame others, staff, patients or their relatives.

11. Consent gained? Record whether it was given and whether it was informed.

12. Make sure that your practice is up to date and matches any changes in hospital policies or procedures, NMC requirements or the law. Saying 'I didn't know' will not hold up in court.

These 12 steps are applicable to any form of patient record or documentation, from completing a record of vital signs or a referral form for a patient, to recording the review of a patient's progress. .

Never assume that information which you have passed to a colleague will be remembered. Don't rely on someone else to complete the records about a patient you have been looking after. You are accountable; losing your registration is a high price to pay for not doing a bit of writing.

This may leave you wondering why you became a nurse; but where would the world be without nurses? The nursing profession is continually striving to improve patient care, and record keeping and documentation are just one aspect of how we are attempting to do this.

What do I need to know about clinical governance?

Flo Brett

'Another jargon term', 'Something meaning nothing', 'Nothing to do with me', 'The latest management talk': are any of these close to your reaction? What is clinical governance? Who is responsible for its implementation? Is it jargon? Will it affect your practice and should you know more about it?

As a staff nurse, my reaction was similar to some of the above, but as I gained more experience and began to understand what clinical governance involved and how it could influence patient care, I started to realise that it was going to help me, not hinder me. So let's explore some of the commonly asked questions regarding clinical governance.

Where did clinical governance come from?

The driving forces behind the clinical governance agenda can be found in the following documents:

- *The New NHS: Modern, Dependable* (Department of Health, 1997), which sets out a modernisation programme to deliver more consistent, higher quality care.

- *A First Class Service: Quality in the new NHS* (Department of Health, 1998), which details a framework for quality improvement outlining clear lines of responsibility and accountability for the overall quality of clinical care.

What is a working definition of clinical governance?

Clinical governance is an umbrella term for all the things that help to maintain and improve high standards of patient care. Clinical governance is not a 'thing', but a framework that is designed to help doctors, nurses and other health professionals to improve clinical standards within the NHS.

Why do I need to know about clinical governance?

- It helps you to deliver safe, up-to-date practice.
- It creates a patient-centred culture, where patients are informed about their care.
- Clinical errors are prevented whenever possible
- Staff treat patients courteously and involve them in decisions.
- Patient services are continuously improved.
- Healthcare professionals are up to date in their practice.

Important aspects of clinical governance

To implement clinical governance, we need to work to promote and support:

- A learning environment.
- An open culture where staff share ideas and experiences within the trust and with others outside the organisation.
- Teamworking where multidisciplinary teams work effectively together.
- Active involvement of patients and carers to inform improvements in our service.

What can I do within my role to help make clinical governance work?

- Have an open mind about new ways of doing things.
- Apply evidence-based standards to your everyday practice – ask why you do things the way you do and what is the evidence to support your decisions.
- Maintain your own professional development.
- Take part in clinical audit within your area.
- Think about ways to improve how you do things, and share ideas with colleagues.
- Talk to colleagues and your manager if you are concerned about standards or practices.

What are my rights and responsibilities regarding risk management?

Paul Rigby

Assessing and managing risk is an important part of the nurse's role and occurs in all arenas of nursing practice. The *Code of Professional Conduct* (NMC, 2004a) outlines clearly the responsibilities that registered nurses have to 'act to identify and minimise the risk to patients and clients'. These are:

- Effective teamworking to promote safe and therapeutic healthcare environments.

- Act quickly to protect patients/clients from risk.

- Where circumstances in the environment cannot be remedied, a report must be made to a senior manager, supported by a written record.

- Have a professional duty to provide safe and competent care.

Risk assessment and risk management

People often confuse the very different concepts of risk assessment and risk management, and a clear understanding of the differences is a useful starting point for any examination of risk.

- **Risk assessment** involves identifying, through the systematic collection of information, and defining what can go wrong in a situation, and predicting and measuring the likelihood of harm occurring.

- **Risk management** is the measures taken to control risks or to minimise their occurrence.

Doyle (1998) has described a cycle of risk management, which can provide a useful frame of reference when considering the management of clinical risk (*Figure 10.1*).

Aims of risk assessment and risk management

Raven (1999) has identified four basic aims of risk assessment/management:

- Protection and safety of the patient/family/community
- Minimising/reducing risk
- Minimising litigation risk (personal/organisational)
- Involvement of the patient/carer in the risk assessment/management process.

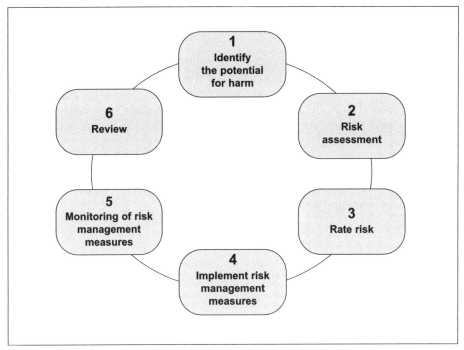

Figure 10.1. Risk management cycle (Doyle, 1998).

While there are an increasing number of clinical risk assessment tools available for the nurse to use, it is important to bear in mind certain principles that accompany the process:

- Clinical risk assessment involves patients and is therefore an interpersonal process.

- Although clinical risk assessment tools can be very useful, you do need to draw from a wide variety of sources for your information.

- Risk assessments should be grounded in history and based upon empirical evidence
- You need to focus upon probability rather than certainty.

- Rather than focusing upon at-risk people, you should focus upon at-risk situations (Ryrie, 2000).

- Risk assessment and risk management responsibilities should be shared within the multiprofessional team.

Effective teamworking and decision making are essential components of successful risk management. Risk management is an ongoing process and the opinions of all team members should be sought on a regular basis. Use reflection and your clinical supervision to seek support, share ideas and solve problems.

Clear, objective and accurate record keeping is an important responsibility for all nurses. To maintain public confidence it is important that practice is seen to be not only professional and evidence based, but also accountable (Department of Health, 2000a). Even if mistakes are made, it is important that the appropriate lessons are learnt and the necessary changes to practice are made.

As a registered nurse, you have a responsibility to highlight deficiencies in training, communication, teamwork and clinical supervision as well as direct patient care; it is important to bear in mind that all of these factors can affect the process of assessing and managing risk.

What else do I need to know?

Personal notes and local contacts

References

Addison R (1999) Practical procedures for nurses No 37.1. Fluid intake and continence care. *Nurs Times* **95**(49): 2-page insert

Agency for Health Care Policy and Prevention (AHCPR) (1992) *Pressure Ulcers in Adults: Prediction and Prevention. Clinical Practice Guideline Number 3.* Department of Health and Human Sciences (now known as Agency of Health Care Research and Quality, AHRQ), Maryland, US

Alderson P (1993) *Children's Consent to Surgery.* Open University Press, Buckingham

Alexander M, Fawcett J, Runciman P (Eds) (2000) *Nursing Practice: Hospital & Home – The Adult.* 2nd edn. Churchill Livingstone, Edinburgh

American College of Surgeons (ACS) (1989) *Advanced Trauma Life Support Manual.* ACS, Chicago

Anderson P (2000) Tickling patients' taste buds. *Nurs Times* **96**(50): 24–26

Andrews M (1996) Using reflection to develop clinical expertise. *Br J Nurs* **5**(8): 508–513

Andrews M, Chilton F (2000) Student and mentor perceptions of mentoring effectiveness. *Nurse Educ Today* **20**(7): 555–562

Association of Medical Microbiologists (1995) Facts about MRSA. Online at: http://www.amm.co.uk

Audit Commission (2001) *A Spoonful of Sugar: Medicines management in NHS hospitals.* Audit Commission, London

Audit Commission (2002) *Review of National Findings: Medicines management.* Audit Commission, London

Baestin AM (1997) Documentation: the reviewer perspective. *Geriatr Rehabil* **13**(1): 14–22

Barton A, Kay S, White G (2000) Managing people on sip feeds in the community. *Br J Community Nurs* **5**(11): 541–547

Beyea SC, Nicoll LH (1996) Administering IM injections the right way. *Am J Nurs* **96**(1): 34–5

Bick C (2000) 'Please help! I'm newly qualified'. *Nurs Stand* **14**(16): 44–47

Bond S (Ed) (1997) *Eating Matters: A resource for improving dietary care in hospitals.* Centre for Health Services Research, Newcastle

Bozeman WP (2001) Shock, Hemorrhagic. Online at: http://www.emedicine.com/emerg/topic 531.htm (last accessed 12.11.03)

Briggs M, Wilson S, Fuller A (1996) The principles of aseptic technique in wound care. *Prof Nurse* **11**(12): 805–808

British Journal of Nursing (2002) One in 10 hospital patients suffer some form of harm. *Br J Nurs* **11**(12): 796

Brykczynska G (1992) Caring – a dying art. In: Jolley M, Brykczynska G (Eds) *Nursing Care: The Challenge to Change.* Edward Arnold, Kent

Bryson E (2001) Drug administration via a nasogastric tube. *Nurs Times* **97**(16): 51
Buckman R (1992) *How to Break Bad News: A guide for healthcare professionals.* Macmillan, London
Burnham P (2000) A guide to nasogastric tube insertion. *Nurs Times* **96**(8 Suppl): 6–7
Burr RG, Nuseibeh IM (1997) Urinary catheter blockage depends on urine pH, calcium and rate of flow. *Spinal Cord* **35**(8): 521–525
Carlisle D (2002) Hidden agenda. *Nurs Times* **98**(21): 24–27
Cavell G (2000) Drugs: the nurse's responsibility. *Prof Nurse* **15**(5): 296
Cavell G, Hughes DK (1997) Does computerised prescribing improve the accuracy of drug administration? *Pharmaceutical Journal* **259**: 782–784
Charnley E (1999) Occupational stress in the newly qualified staff nurse. *Nurs Stand* **13**(29): 33–36
Clarke M (2002) Pressure-redistribution cushions: the Cinderella of support surfaces? *Nurs Times* **98**(8 Suppl): 59–60
Cohen SS (2003) *Trauma Nursing Secrets.* Hanley & Belfus Inc, Philadelphia: 109–114
Colagiovanni L (2000) Preventing and clearing blocked feeding tubes. *Nurs Times* **96** (17 Suppl): 3–4
Colley W (1998) Practical Procedures for Nurses No 8. Continence assessment. *Nurs Times* **94**(6): 2-page insert
Collins J (1988) Should doctors tell the truth? In: Callaghan J (Ed). *Ethical Issues in Modern Medicine.* Oxford University Press, Oxford
Collins T (2000) Understanding shock. *Nurs Stand* **14**(49): 35–39
Cook M, Hale C, Watson B (1999) Interrater reliability and the assessment of pressure-sore risk using an adapted Waterlow Scale. *Clinical Effectiveness in Nursing* **3**: 66–74
Cooke H (2000) *When Someone Dies: A practical guide to holistic care at the end of life.* Butterworth-Heinemann, Oxford
Costello J, Trinder-Brook A (2000) Children's nurses' experience of caring for dying children in hospital. *Paediatr Nurs* **12**: 6
Courtenay M, Butler M (2002) Education and nurse prescribing. *Nurs Times* **98**(9): 53–54
Coyle N (1986) Continuous subcutaneous infusions of opiates in cancer patients with pain. *Oncol Nurs Forum* **13**(4): 53–57
Crow S (1989) Asepsis – an indispensable part of the patient's care plan. *Crit Care Nurs Q* **11**(4): 11–16
Daloz LA (1986) *Effective Teaching and Mentoring.* Jossey-Bass, San Francisco
Deakin CD, Low JL (2000) Accuracy of the advanced trauma life support guidelines for predicting systolic blood pressure using carotid, femoral and radial pulses: observational study. *BMJ* **321**(7262): 673–674
Department of Health (1994) *Being Heard: The report of a review committee on NHS complaints procedures (Wilson Report).* HMSO, London
Department of Health (1996) MRSA – what nursing and residential homes need to know. Online at: http://www.dh.gov.uk/Home/fs/en
Department of Health (1997) *The New NHS: Modern, Dependable.* Cm 3807. The Stationery Office, London
Department of Health (1998) *A First Class Service: Quality in the new NHS.* The

Stationery Office, London

Department of Health (1999a) *Making a Difference: Strengthening the nursing, midwifery and health visiting contribution to health and healthcare* (The Crown Report). HMSO, London

Department of Health (1999b) *Review of Prescribing, Supply and Administration of Medicines. Final report.* HMSO, London

Department of Health (2000a) *An Organisation with a Memory: Report of an expert group on learning from adverse events in the NHS.* The Stationery Office, London

Department of Health (2000b) *Patient Group Directions (England only).* HSC2000/026. Health & Safety Commission, London

Department of Health (2000c) *The NHS Plan: A plan for investment, a plan for reform.* Cm 4818-I. The Stationery Office, London

Department of Health (2000d) *A Health Service of All the Talents: Developing the NHS workforce.* Consultation document on the review of workforce planning. NHS Executive, Leeds

Department of Health (2001a) *The Essence of Care: Patient-focused benchmarking for health care practitioners.* DH, London

Department of Health (2001b) *Seeking Consent: Working with children.* DH, London

Department of Health (2001c) *Good Practice in Consent Implementation Guide: Consent to examination or treatment.* DH, London

Department of Health (2001d) *Reference Guide to Consent for Examination or Treatment.* DH, London

Department of Health (2001e) Patients to get quicker access to medicines. Press release 4.5.2001 Ref. 2001/0223

Department of Health (2001f) *Building a Safer NHS for Patients: Implementing an organisation with a memory.* DH, London

Department of Health and Welsh Office (1999) *Code of Practice: Mental Health Act 1983.* The Stationery Office, London

Dimond B (2002) Workplace stress and bullying: liabilities of the employer. *Br J Nurs* **11**(10) 699–701

Dimond B (2004) *Legal Aspects of Nursing.* 4th edn. Prentice Hall, New York

Dimond B, Barker F (1996) *Mental Health Law for Nurses.* Blackwell Science, Oxford

Dougherty S, Simmons R (1992) The biology and practice of surgical drainage. Part 1. *Curr Probl Surg* **29**(8): 559–623

Dowse J, MacKender J (2000) Back to basics: continence. *Nurs Times* **96**(30 Suppl): 7–9

Doyle M (1998) Clinical risk assessment for mental health nurses. *Nurs Times* **94**(17): 47–49

Doyle M, Hanks G, Chery N, Calman K (Eds) (2003) *Oxford Textbook of Palliative Medicine.* 3rd edn. Oxford University Press, Oxford

Edwards S (2001) Shock: types, classifications and explorations of their physiological effects. *Emerg Nurse* **9**(2): 29–38

Ellis H (1997) *Clinical Anatomy: A revision and applied anatomy for clinical students.* 9th edn. Blackwell Science, Oxford: 333

English National Board for Nursing, Midwifery and Health Visiting (2001a) *Placements in Focus: Guidance for education in practice for health care professions.* ENB, London

English National Board for Nursing, Midwifery and Health Visiting (2001b) *Preparation of Mentors and Teachers: A new framework for guidance.* ENB, London

Evans A, Godfrey H (2001) Bladder washouts in the management of long-term catheters. In: Pope Cruickshank J, Woodward S (Eds) *Management of Continence and Urinary Catheter Care.* BJN Monograph. Quay Books, Dinton, Wiltshire

Evans K (2001) Expectations of newly qualified nurses. *Nurs Stand* **15**(41): 33–38

Faull R, Woof R (2002) *Palliative Care.* Oxford University Press, Oxford

Fortes Mayer K (2002) The process of obtaining informed patient consent. *Nurs Times* **98**(31): 30–31

Fowler J (Ed) (1999) *The Handbook of Clinical Supervision.* Quay Books, Dinton, Wiltshire

Fulton GB, Metress EK (1995) *Perspectives on Death and Dying.* Jones and Bartlett Publishers, Boston, US

Galford J (1990) *Nursing Calculations.* 3rd edn. Churchill Livingstone, Edinburgh

Garnham P (2001) Understanding and dealing with anger, aggression and violence. *Nurs Stand* **16**(6): 37–42

Gates A (2000) The benefits of irrigation in catheter care. *Prof Nurse* **16**(1): 835–838

Geary M (2000) PHCP 2052/3052: Symptom control in palliative and terminal care. (Unpublished paper). De Montfort University, Leicester

Gebhardt K (2002) Pressure ulcer prevention. Part 3. Prevention strategies. *Nurs Times* **98**(13): 37–40

General Medical Council (2002) Referring a doctor to the GMC: Guidance for members of the medical profession and other healthcare professionals. Online at: http://www.gmc-uk.org/probdocs/default.htm (accessed 20/02/2005)

Gibbs G (1988) *Learning by Doing: A guide to teaching and learning methods.* Further Education Unit, Oxford Brookes University, Oxford

Gilsenan I (2000) A practical guide to giving injections. *Nurs Times* **96**(33): 43–44

Godfrey H, Evans A (2001) Catherisation and urinary tract infections microbiology. In: Pope Cruickshank J, Woodward S (2001) *Management of Continence and Urinary Catheter Care.* BJN Monograph. Quay Books, Dinton, Wiltshire

Goodinson SM (1986a) Fundamentals of drug action administration and absorption: an overview. *Nursing (Lond)* **3**(10): 386–390

Goodinson SM (1986b) Fundamentals of drug action: drug elimination. *Nursing (Lond)* **3**(12): 466–467

Gray MA, Smith LN (2000) The qualities of an effective mentor from the student nurse's perspective: findings from a longitudinal qualitative study. *J Adv Nurs* **32**(6): 1542–1549

Grayless R, Martin S, Markevics M (2002) Using a wound care formulary to raise nursing standards. *Nurs Times* **98**(2): 49–52

Green C (2001) Benefiting from the end of blame culture. *Prof Nurse* **16**(7 Suppl): S3–S4

Green S (2000) Oral dietary supplements. *J Community Nurs* **14**(3): 26–28

Grove J (2000) Survival and resistance. *Nurs Times* **96**(18): 26–28

Guy H (2004) Preventing pressure ulcers: choosing a mattress. *Prof Nurse* **20**(4): 43–46

Haddock J, Bassett C (1997) Nurses' perceptions of reflective practice. *Nurs Stand* **11**(32): 39–41

Hand H (2001) Shock. *Nurs Stand* **15**(48): 45–52
Hatchett R (2000) Central venous pressure measurements. *Nurs Times* **96**(15): 49–50
Health Service Ombudsman for England (2002) *Annual Report 2001–2002*. HMSO, London
Health Which? (1999) Blowing the whistle. *Health Which?* April: 16–17
Herth K (1990) Fostering hope in terminally ill people. *J Adv Nurs* **15**: 1520–1529
Higgins D (2002a) Breaking bad news in cancer care. *Prof Nurse* **17**(10): 609
Hindle T (1998) *Reducing Stress*. Dorling Kindersley, London
Horan D, Coad J (2000) Can nurses improve patient feeding? *Nurs Times* **96**(50): 33–34
Howell M (2002) Do nurses know enough about percutaneous endoscopic gastrostomy? *Nurs Times* **98**(17): 40–42
Howells-Johnson J (2000) Verbal abuse. *Br J Perioper Nurs* **10**(10): 508–511
Hulatt I (1995) A sad reflection. *Nurs Stand* **9**(20): 22–23
Jackson J (2001) *Truth, Trust and Medicine*. Routledge, London
Jarvis P (1992) Reflective practice and nursing. *Nurse Educ Today* **12**(3): 174–181
Jarvis P, Gibson S (Eds) (1997) *The Teacher Practitioner and Mentor in Nursing, Midwifery and Health Visiting and the Social Services*. 2nd edn. Stanley Thornes, Cheltenham
Jassal S (2001) Basic symptom control in paediatric palliative care. Unpublished guidelines, 3rd edn. The Rainbows Children's Hospice, Loughborough, Leicestershire
Jevon P (2002) *Advanced Cardiac Life Support: A practical guide*. Butterworth-Heinemann, Oxford
John A, Stevenson T (1995) A basic guide to the principles of drug therapy. *Br J Nurs* **4**(20): 1194–1198
Johns C (2000) *Becoming a Reflective Practitioner*. Blackwell Science, London
Jones G (2003) Care of the emergency patient – frameworks for nursing assessment and management. In: Jones G, Endacott R, Crouch R (Eds) *Emergency Nursing Care: Principles and Practice*. Greenwich Medical Media, London: 9-26
Kaye P (1992) *A to Z of Hospice and Palliative Medicine*. EPL Publications, Northampton
Kelly J (2001) Minimising potential side-effects of medication at different ages. *Prof Nurse* **17**(4): 259–262
Kern K, Hilwig R, Berg R, Ewy G (1998) Efficacy of chest compression-only BLS CPR in the presence of an occluded airway. *Resuscitation* **39**(3); 179–188
Knowles M (1973) *The Adult Learner: A neglected species*. 1st edn. Gulf Publishing Company, Houston, Texas
Knowles M (1980) *The Modern Practice of Adult Education: From Pedagogy to Andragogy*. Follett, Chicago, Illinois
Kolecki P (2001) Shock, Hypovolaemic. Online at: http://www.emedicine.com/EMERG/topic532.htm (accessed 12.11.03)
Kubler-Ross E (1970) *On Death and Dying: Care of the patient, relatives/carers following a death*. Tavistock/Routledge, London
Lathlean J (1987) Are you prepared to be a staff nurse? *Nurs Times* **83**(36): 25–27
Laurent C (1998) Catheters: making the right choice. *Nurs Times* **94**(25) 64–66
Lavender R (2000) Cranberry juice: the facts. *Nurs Times* **96**(40 Suppl): 11–12
Leaver R (1996) Cranberry juice: therapeutic uses in urinary tract disorders. *Prof Nurse* **11**(8): 525–526

Leadbeater M (1991) Increasing knowledge. *Nurs Times* **87**(30): 32–35

Lloyd Jones M, Walters S, Akehurst R (2001) The implications of contact with the mentor for preregistration nursing and midwifery students. *J Adv Nurs* **35**(2): 151–160

Maki D, Ringer M (1987) Evaluation of dressing regimens for the prevention of infection with peripheral intravenous catheters. Gauze, a transparent polyurethane dressing, and an iodophor-transparent dressing. *JAMA* **258**(17): 2396–2403

Mallett J, Dougherty L (Eds) (2000) *The Royal Marsden Hospital Manual of Clinical Nursing Procedures.* 5th edn. Blackwell Science, Oxford

Martin V (2000) Managing your time. Part 3. *Nurs Times* **96**(18): 42

Maslow AH (1943) A theory of human motivation. *Psychology Review* **50**: 370–396

McCaffery M (1968) Nursing practice theories related to cognition, bodily pain, and man-environment interactions. University of California at Los Angeles Students' Store

McCormac M (1990) Managing hemorrhagic shock. *Am J Nurs* **90**(8): 22–27

McGill S (1982) Catheter management: it's the size that's important. *Nurs Mirror* **154**(14): 48–49

McLaren S, Holmes S, Bond S (1997) Section 3: The evidence about eating and nutritional needs. In: Bond S. *A Resource for Improving Dietary Care in Hospitals.* Centre for Health Services Research, Newcastle

McSherry R, Kell J, Pearce P (2002) Clinical supervision and clinical governance. *Nurs Times* **98**(23): 30–32

Mooney G, Comerford D (2003) What you need to know about central venous lines. *Nurs Times* **99**(10): 28–29

Morton-Cooper A, Palmer A (1993) *Mentoring, Preceptorship and Clinical Supervision: A guide to professional roles in clinical practice.* 2nd edn. Blackwell Science, Oxford

Mosby's Medical, Nursing and Allied Health Dictionary (2002) 6th edn. Mosby, St Louis

Moulton C, Yates D (1999) *Lecture Notes on Emergency Medicine.* 2nd edn. Blackwell Science, Oxford: 175

National Institute for Clinical Excellence (2001) *Pressure Ulcer Risk Assessment and Prevention.* Inherited Clinical Guideline B. NICE, London

Nazarko L (1995) The therapeutic uses of cranberry juice. *Nurs Stand* **9**(34): 33–35

Nazarko L (1998) Breaking the silence. *Elder Care* **10**(3): 44

Nichol M, Bavin C, Bedford-Turner S, Cronin P, Rawlings-Anderson K (2000) *Essential Nursing Skills.* Mosby, London

Nicholson H (1986) The success of the syringe driver. *Nurs Times* **82**(28): 49–51

Nursing & Midwifery Council (2002) *Supporting Nurses and Midwives through Lifelong Learning.* NMC, London

Nursing & Midwifery Council (2003) Professional Conduct FAQs. http://www.nmc-uk.org/nmc/main/advice/professionalConductFaqs.html (accessed 20/02/2005)

Nursing & Midwifery Council (2004a) *Code of Professional Conduct.* NMC, London

Nursing & Midwifery Council (2004b) *Complaints about Unfitness to Practise: A guide for members of the Public.* NMC, London

Nursing & Midwifery Council (2004c) *Guidelines for the Administration of Medicines.* NMC, London

Nursing & Midwifery Council (2004d) *The PREP Handbook.* NMC, London

Nursing & Midwifery Council (2004e) *Guidelines for Records and Record Keeping.* NMC, London

Nursing Times (1994a) Professional development. Medication: knowledge for practice. *Nurs Times* **90**(36 Suppl): 1–4

Nursing Times (1994b) Professional development. Medication: the role of the nurse. *Nurs Times* **90**(37 Suppl): 5–8

O'Dowd A (2002) Is legislation protecting nurses who blow the whistle? *Nurs Times* **98**(46): 10–11

O'Reilly M (2003) Major trauma management. In: Jones G, Endacott R, Crouch R (Eds). *Emergency Nursing Care: Principles and Practice.* Greenwich Medical Media Limited. London: 105–134

Pearce L (2001) Bully at work. *Nurs Stand* **15**(27): 14–15

Pomfret I (1999) Catheter care – trouble shooting. *J Community Nurs* **13**(6): 20–24

Power K (1996) First time practice as a children's nurse: a phenomenological inquiry. Unpublished dissertation. De Montfort University, Leicester

Prescribing Nurse Bulletin (1999) Vol 1, pp 2-3. National Prescribing Centre, London

Public Concern at Work (2002) Whistleblowing dos and don'ts. Online at: http://www.pcaw.co.uk/help_individ/dos_donts.html (accessed 13/02/2003)

Raven J (1999) Managing the unmanageable: risk assessment and risk management in contemporary professional practice. *J Nurs Manag* **7**(4): 201–206

Reed S, Hambridge K, Land L (2001) Implementing best practice in pressure ulcer prevention. *Nurs Times NT Plus Suppl* **97**(24): 69–71

Regnaud C (2004) Dysphagia, dyspepsia and hiccup. In: Doyle D *et al* (Eds) *Oxford Textbook of Palliative Medicine.* New York: Oxford University Press, New York: 468–483

Resuscitation Council (UK) (2000a) *Basic Life Support Resuscitation Guidelines.* Resuscitation Council, London

Resuscitation Council (UK) (2000b) *Cardiopulmonary Resuscitation: Guidance for Clinical Practice and Training in Hospitals.* Resuscitation Council, London

Resuscitation Council (UK) (2001) *Cardiopulmonary Resuscitation: Guidance for Clinical Practice and Training in Primary Care.* Resuscitation Council, London

Resuscitation Council (UK) (2002) *Immediate Life Support Manual.* Resuscitation Council London

Rew M (2001) Use of catheter maintenance solutions for long-term catheters. In: Pope Cruickshank J, Woodward S (Eds). *Management of Continence and Urinary Catheter Care.* BJN Monograph. Quay Books, Dinton, Wiltshire

Rew M, Woodward S (2001) Troubleshooting common problems associated with long-term urinary catheters. In: Pope Cruickshank J, Woodward S. *Management of Continence and Urinary Catheter Care.* British Journal of Nursing Monograph. Quay Books, Dinton, Wiltshire

Rice V (1991) Shock, a clinical syndrome: an update. Part 1. An overview of shock. *Crit Care Nurse* **11**(4): 20–24, 26–27

Robotham M (2001) How to handle complaints. *Nurs Times* **97**(30): 25–28

Royal College of Nursing (2001) *Clinical Practice Guidelines. Pressure Ulcer Risk Assessment and Prevention – Recommendations.* RCN, London

Royal College of Nursing (2002) Whistleblowing. Online at:

http://www.rcn.org.uk/rcn_extranet/rcn_direct/Display.php3?BSID=318 (accessed 13/02/2003)

Rudd N (2002) *A Guide to Prescribing for Patients with Advanced Malignancy*. Leicestershire Cancer Centre, Leicester

Russell L (1999) The importance of wound documentation and classification. *Br J Nurs* **8**(20): 1342–1343, 1346, 1348 passim

Ryrie I (2000) Assessing risk. In: Gamble C, Brennan G (Eds). *Working with Serious Mental Illness: A manual for clinical practice*. Baillière Tindall/RCN, London

Shand M (1987) Unreasonable expectations? *Nurs Times* **83**(36): 28–30

Sheff B (2003) Multidrug-resistant microorganisms: still making waves. *Nursing* **33**(11): 59–64

Shepherd M (2002a) Medicines 1. Pharmacology. *Nurs Times* **98**(15): 43–46

Shepherd M (2002b) Administration of medicines. *Nurs Times* **98**(16): 45–48

Shepherd M (2002c) Managing medicines. *Nurs Times* **98**(17): 43–46

Smith L, Baker F, McDougall C, Stead L (1999) Removal of a vacuum drain. *Nurs Times* **95**(11 Suppl): 1–2

Snowball R (1999) Finding the evidence: an information skills approach. In: Dawes M, Davies P, Gray A, Mant J et al. *Evidence Based Practice: A primer for health care professionals*. Churchill Livingstone, Edinburgh

Speechley V, Toovey J (1987) Problems in IV therapy. *Prof Nurse* **2**(8): 240–242

Spouse J (1996) The effective mentor: a model for student-centred learning. *Nurs Times* **92**(13): 32–35

Spyropoulos A (2002) Patient group directions. *Nurs Times* **98**(9): 48

Stewart E (2001) Urinary catheters: selection, maintenance and nursing care. In: Pope Cruickshank J, Woodward S (Eds) (2001) *Management of Continence and Urinary Catheter Care*. BJN Monograph. Quay Books, Dinton, Wiltshire

Stickler DJ, Zimakoff J (1994) Complications of urinary tract infections associated with devices used for long-term bladder management. *J Hosp Infect* **28**(3): 177–194

Strachan I (2001) Medicines and older people: a nurse's guide to administration. *Br J Community Nurs* **6**(6): 296–301

Thomas HDG (2001) *Law Study Notes*. Quantum Development (www.quantum-development.co.uk/criticalcare.htm)

Torrance C, Maylor M (1999) Pressure sore survey: part one. *Journal of Wound Care* **8**(1): 27-30

Treloar A, Beats B, Philpot M (2000) A pill in the sandwich: covert medication in food and drink. *J R Soc Med* **93**(8): 408–411

Treloar A, Philpot M, Beats B (2001) Concealing medicines in patient's food. *Lancet* **357**(9249): 62–64

Turner T (1985) Which dressing and why? In: Westaby S (Ed). *Wound Care*. William Heinemann, London

Twycross R (2002) *Introducing Palliative Care*. 4th edn. Radcliffe Medical Press, Abingdon

Twycross R, Wilcock A (2001) *Symptom Management in Advanced Cancer*. Radcliffe Medical Press, Abingdon

United Kingdom Central Council for Nursing, Midwifery and Health Visiting (1986) *Administration of Medicines Advisory Paper*. UKCC, London

United Kingdom Central Council for Nursing, Midwifery and Health Visiting (1994)

The Council's Standards for Education and Practice following Registration: Programmes leading to the Qualification of Specialist Practitioner. UKCC, London

United Kingdom Central Council for Nursing, Midwifery and Health Visiting (2001) *UKCC Position Statement on the Covert Administration of Medicines: Disguising medicine in food and drink*. UKCC, London

University Hospitals of Leicester Nutrition Support Team (2002) Insertion of a nasogastric tube policy. UHL NHS Trust. Unpublished

Van Belkum A, Verbrugh H (2001) 40 years of methicillin resistant *Staphylococcus aureus*. *BMJ* **323**(7314): 645–646

Wallis L (2001) Protecting the whistleblower. *Nurs Stand* **13**(47): 16–17

Walsh M (Ed) (2003) *Watson's Clinical Nursing and Related Sciences*. 6th edn. Baillière Tindall, London

Wells M (1998) Coping with common catheter care problems. *Community Nurse* **4**(3): 22–24

Wheeler J (2001) Staff development through appraisal. *Nurs Times* **97**(39): 34

White C (2002a) The enemy within. *Nurs Times* **98**(44): 12–13

White C (2002b) Furniture is harbouring superbugs, says study. *Nurs Times* **98**(22): 7

Wiechula R, Hodgkinson B (2002) *Promoting Best Practice in the Management of Peripheral Intravascular Devices*. Evaluation Cycle Report No. 2. The Joanna Briggs Institute for Evidence Based Nursing & Midwifery, Royal Adelaide Hospital, Australia. http://www.joannabriggs.edu.au/pdf/evaliv.pdf (last accessed 6 June 2005)

Williams B (1991) Medication education. *Nurs Times* **87**(29): 50–52

Winn C (1998) Complications with urinary catheters. *Prof Nurse* **13**(Suppl 5): 7–10

World Health Organization (1996) *Cancer Pain Relief: With a guide to opioid availability*. WHO, Geneva

Workman B (1999) Safe injection techniques. *Nurs Stand* **13**(39): 47–53

Worthington KA (2002) Hazardous drugs. *Am J Nurs* **102**(5): 120

Wyatt PJ, Illingworth RN, Clancy MJ, Munro P, Robertson CE (1999) *Oxford Handbook of Accident and Emergency Medicine*. Oxford University Press, Oxford: 122–124, 126, 164–173, 578, 602, 610–616

Index

A

action plan 59
advanced standing 150
aggression 25–26
agonists 84
airway obstruction 1–3
alginates 55
analgesia 52, 166
analgesic three-step ladder 167
accreditation of prior achievement (APA) 148, 150
accreditation of prior experiential learning (APEL) 150
adverse reactions 89
aseptic technique 47, 57
assessment 5, 39, 48, 56, 61–62, 125–129
~ formative 120–122
~ of achievement of nursing competence 115
~ of breathing 5
~ of nutritional status 70
~ of pressure ulcer risk 66
~ of students 117–118
assessors 115–116

B

bacteria 34, 55–56, 65
basic life support 4–9
benchmarking 39
bereavement 160
blood loss 3, 11–15, 17–18
blood pressure 11–14
bullying 31–33

C

cancer 41, 166
cannula 16, 45–47, 52
cardiac abnormalities 2
cardiac arrest 1–3
cardiorespiratory arrest 1, 3–4, 9–10
credit accumulation and transfer (CAT) points 148, 150
catheter care 47
catheterisation 18, 39, 47–50, 65
chest compressions 7-8, 10
clinical experience 145
clinical governance 184–185
clinical supervision 140, 145–147, 154
community services 73-74
compensatory stage 11–14
complaints 23–25
consent 43, 49, 51, 53–54, 60–61, 63, 67, 180–181
constipation 70, 157, 173
continence 39, 64–65, 173

D

death 10, 12
~ contacting relatives following 158
degree 149
dehydration 45, 67
professional practice 145
diarrhoea 45, 70, 162
dietitians 75
difficult questions 21
drug administration 79, 44, 63
~ ethical issues in 106
~ intravenous 105

~ nurse's role in 79
~ oral 101
~ parenteral 104
~ rectal 102
~ sublingual 102
~ topical 103
drug distribution 83
dyspnoea 157, 162, 174

E

evaluation 39, 68

F

feedback 117, 119–121, 126–129
first impressions 127
fluid resuscitation 15–16, 18
foams 55, 68

G

gastrostomy 44, 70
discharging patients 73, 75–76
grief 160

H

haemorrhage 1, 10–17
halo effect 127
handwashing 35–36
healthcare assistants 134
hydrocolloids 55
hydrofibres 55
hydrogels 55

I

incident reporting 21, 27
infection control team 35
infusion sites
~ selection of 52

interviews 153
intestinal obstruction 172
intravenous therapy 39, 45
investigations 39, 48, 58–64
~ preparing patients for 58
iodine–based products 56
IV fluid 16

L

larval therapy 56
last offices 163
learning environment 123
learning outcomes 122
learning resources 124
legal and professional frameworks 80

M

malnourished 69–70
malpractice 29–31, 33
Medicines Act 1968 80
mentors 115–120
Mental Health Act 179
methicillin–resistant *Staphylococcus aureus* (MRSA) 34–36
Misuse of Drugs Act 1971 80

N

National Institute for Clinical Effectiveness (NICE) 81
National Service Frameworks 81
nasogastric tube 42–44
nausea 70, 169
nurse prescribing 79, 112
Nurse Prescribing Act 1992 81

O

occupational therapists 75
opioids 168

oral thrush 175

P

pain assessment 166
pain 160, 164, 166
palliative care 157
partial agonists 84
paste bandages 56
patient group directions 111
personal professional profile 142–143
pharmacology 79, 83
physiotherapists 75
podiatrists 76
post–registration education and practice (PREP) 142
pressure ulcers 66–69
prioritisation 132, 137–138
professional development 140, 142–146, 149
professional misconduct 29
Public Interest Disclosure Act 1998 30, 33

R

record keeping 62, 182–183
referring patients 74–76
~ to multidisciplinary team 75
~ to specialist nurses 76
reflection 62
reflective practice 151
relatives 157
research 146
research process 137, 140, 146
respiratory arrest 3
risk management 186–188

S

secondment 146
self–discharge 33–34
shift work 139–140

shock 3, 10–12, 15, 18
~ haepovolaemic 11
silver–based products 56
special duty payments 139
specialist nurses 73–74, 76
specimens 62–63
speech therapists 76
stereotyping 127
supervisors 115–116, 121
symptom control 162
syringe drivers 52, 170, 172

T

team 9–10, 18, 131–133
terminally ill 48
terminally ill, the 175–176
terminally ill child 161
time management 132, 137–138
tulles 56

U

university 120
unsocial hours, working 139
urinary tract 39, 65
urinary tract infection 39, 65

V

VAC therapy 56
validated programmes 146
vapour–permeable films 55
ventilation 3, 6, 9, 15–16
vomiting 42, 45, 70

W

ward rounds 134
wound drains 40–41
wound dressings 39, 54–56
wound manager bags 56